The

Balance

The
Balance

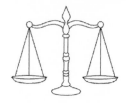

Divine and
Natural Healing,
Health, and Thorns

Shaun Eller

The Balance
Copyright © 2019
Shaun Eller

Unless otherwise noted, all Scripture quotations herein are from the Authorized King James Version of the Bible.

Cover image - Allan Swart © 123RF.com

FOR INFORMATION CONTACT:

Shaun Eller
Seller670@gmail.com
330-418-6255

Acknowledgments

I have had a blessed life. God has been far better to me than I deserve and has surrounded me by incredible people. God gets all the glory for any good that may result from my life. Any gifts, abilities, or opportunities I have came from Him. Thanks be to God because I am nothing without Him.

Thanks to my mentors and pastors. Mr. William Small was a high-school teacher who had a very positive influence on me. I learned a lot from him and have found value from staying in touch with him throughout my life. Pastor F. J. and Rose Ellis have been my pastors since I was eight years old. He is also my father-in-law. He put Angela and me in leadership classes as pre-teenagers. He is passionate about souls and founded a ministry training course, Purpose Institute. My wife and I were in the first graduating class, and the organization has grown into a worldwide ministry training tool that continues to expand. Much of who I am has come from him. After resigning from the pastorate in Canton, we attended The Apostolic Church of Barberton for a few years and sat under the ministry of Rod and Nan Pamer. They are some of the greatest people on earth, and we were privileged to get to know them and serve under them. Nan was also one of the first to read this manuscript and provide pages of feedback to make it better. We spent several years in Pearland, Texas, under Pastor Ken and Tessie Gurley. Pastor Gurley is one of the most creative and anointed orators I have heard, and I was amazed at his engaging and anointed delivery every week. After moving back to Ohio, we have been able to spend time in Barberton but have been working primarily with my brother- and sister-in-law, Joe and Hirma Ellis. Pastor Ellis is a preacher of preachers and a tremendously anointed man of God. All of these influenced our lives, and we are grateful.

I have been blessed to have a great family as well. My parents have given me every opportunity to be successful in life. As a young child, I told my dad I could not decide if I wanted to be a truck driver or a preacher. He asked me to sit and talk with him about it. After some time, we concluded that I should drive a truck and have the back equipped as a church. Thus, I could be a truck driver and a preacher. His wisdom walked me through the journey toward my dreams; he never discouraged me. My mom has always been a consistent prayer warrior. I remember coming from my room in the morning often and seeing her Bible beside the chair where she prayed and read in that morning. I thank her for her prayers. My sister and I had an adversarial relationship in youth, but it transitioned in adulthood. For many years she was my secretary at the Canton church and a huge blessing to the kingdom of God. Since I grew up around my wife, I also grew up with my brothers-in-law. Tom and Joe Ellis are both awesome preachers and great men of God. I have been blessed to grow up with them and to count them, then and now, among my friends.

Finally, I cannot thank God enough for the wonderful wife and children He has given me. My wife has been a huge help in keeping me healthy and has been my best friend since we were eight years old. I am blessed beyond measure and much more than I deserve to have her by my side always. Ellis, Allissa, Elijah, and Israel are among God's greatest blessings. Nothing can bring more joy or pain than being a parent. Elijah has been writing a book while I have been writing this one. About once a month, we go to Panera and work on our books together. I have loved going through this process with him. I am proud of all four children and thank God for allowing me to be their dad.

Contents

Preface

I currently reside in North Canton, Ohio, with my wife and three of our four children. The first thirty-eight years of my life took place in Canton, Ohio. For the next seven years we lived in Pearland, Texas, after my company transferred me to the Houston area. We then moved back to Ohio when I was relocated again to the Canton area for a new position.

In my childhood, my family devoutly adhered to Catholicism. However, when I was eight years old, my father spoke in tongues while in a meeting in the Catholic church. They told him that they did not want anything to do with people speaking in tongues. He met my future father-in-law when he went door to door to invite people to the church he had started in Canton. I grew up in that church and eventually became the youth pastor and then the lead pastor.

This book is really an accumulation of what I have learned, read, and experienced through the years. I have much work to do, but I have been able to combine my life lessons and experiences to find a balance in my life. Balance between a relationship with God and healthy living is not always easy, but if we can live a balanced life, it will allow us to be more productive in the work of God and to enjoy our life to the fullest as we give the kingdom of God our best.

This book was born from a number of situations that happened in my life in the autumn of 2005. The first thoughts came from an article written by J. Mark Jordan, entitled "Thorns have Roses," and published in the June 2005 edition of the *Ohio Apostolic News*. While reading that article I felt God speak, instructing me to preach a message entitled "The Balance." I scheduled the message for October 23, 2005, and filed the article with some of my thoughts on the subject.

A number of unique circumstances occurred in the interval before I preached this message, including some great messages on faith, the death of a young mother in the church from cancer, and a stroke suffered by a guest minister right after he preached a powerful message on faith in our Sunday morning service. As Mary in the Bible "kept all these things, and pondered them in her heart," I did the same and began the development of the process that led to the writing of this book.

These circumstances led to many questions. How could he have a stroke when he just ministered about healing? Why didn't God miraculously heal him like He had healed him previously? Why are times like this the hardest in which to hear from God? Where does healthy eating and a healthy lifestyle fit in with divine healing? What is the fine line between natural healing, divine healing, and medical intervention? When is an affliction a thorn that we have to deal with, and when do we just need more faith for God to do a miracle? Why did God stop the stroke after it started (the doctors said the stroke stopped soon after it started) instead of not allowing it to start? Was it a divine healing that the stroke did not continue, or was that nature?

The bottom line is that we had some guest preachers deliver a couple of powerful messages on healing in just over a month. Meanwhile, in that time we had a funeral of a young mother who died of cancer at the age of thirty-one, and one of our guest speakers had a stroke on the way home from service.

We read Paul's account of a thorn that God chose not to remove and we know that healthy eating is important, but how do we find the balance in all these complex situations? That is what this book is all about.

I have to confess I absolutely love Big Macs, Long John Silvers, and milkshakes of just about any variety. Ice cream is an incredible invention, and while I lived in Texas, the power of Blue Bell made an impact on me. With all that said it has been years since I had a Big Mac. Not that I don't want one, but I know I have to stay away from them. I occasionally have a milkshake and I have probably had LJS once a year if that, but I realize they have to be the exceptions and not the rule. Some days I am too tired to get up and exercise, but that also has to be the exception and not the rule. While I do not agree with everything said by the authors or experts cited in this book, I have gleaned helpful tips from them.

This is a compilation of a lifetime of reading, studying, and living, trying to find the balance. As an assistant coach for our son's football team, I heard another coach close every practice by reciting a Vince Lombardi: quote: "Perfection is not attainable, but if we chase perfection, we can catch excellence." Mr. Lombardi also said, "We didn't lose the game; we just ran out of time." My prayer is that the readers of this book will chase balance, and in the process they won't run out of time but will have fought a good fight, finished the course, and kept the faith in the most balanced, blessed, and abundant life possible.

The Balance

Divine and natural healing – Our bodies usually heal themselves. Healing is the norm, not the exception. There is also the aspect of divine healing. Jesus did this often during His earthly ministry, but He could not do much in His hometown. Since the Scriptures tell us He designated someone to care for His mother as He was on the cross, His earthly father probably died while He was still alive. So sometimes divine healing doesn't happen.

Health – I recently heard about a guy who ate McDonald's extra-value meals three times a day for thirty days. After this experiment about half of his body's functions shut down. Some things I think even God stays away from. Can He heal in these situations? Of course He can. He is God, after all, but He also gave us a brain so we can exercise common sense. He also established some diet restrictions in the Old Testament that give us sensible and practical guidelines.

Thorns – If Paul, the great Christian, apostle, and author of most of the New Testament, was given a thorn,

I don't think we are above having them as well. How do you know the difference between a thorn that God gives and something for which to keep praying for healing? How do we deal with these thorns so we can say as Paul did, "Therefore will I rather glory in my infirmities, that the power of Christ may rest upon me" (2 Corinthians 12:9)? One thing is certain, though. As Paul's pain increased, so did God's grace.

Mental illness – Mental illness introduces another dynamic altogether. Understanding mental illness is very hard, and most of the time we run in the opposite direction when we have to deal with this issue. How should the Christian address the sensitive subject of mental illness in this society where more than 13 percent of the population take antidepressants?

Finances – The pressure to look and live a certain way is consuming. Too often our ideal lifestyle exceeds our income, creates major strain on relationships, and even affects our health. How do we balance finances and lifestyle in our search for a balanced life?

To become – God gives us the power to become what He wants us to be.

As you journey through the pages of this book, we will endeavor to find the answers to some of these perplexing questions. It is my prayer that you will find not only the answers but also some practical knowledge you can apply to help you live a productive, healthy lifestyle that makes your future one to look forward to.

God bless,
Shaun Eller

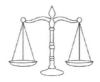

Chapter One

The Balanced Life

The word "balance" is often used among Christian circles, but the problem is that it is frequently misused. People talk about the need for balance between ministry, family, church, and work. We consider these often very contrary ideas as needing balance in our lives.

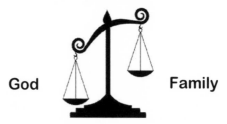

I understand the thoughts behind such ideas, but ultimately all our relationships should be centered around our relationship with God. The solution isn't balancing family on one side of a scale and church on the other but is more accurately displayed as concentric circles, where God is the center of all we do and are.

Rather than opposing one another, the areas of our lives should find a place more like below, where all we do revolves around God. Yet we have to hold some commitments as more important than others. This is why being unequally yoked to another (2 Corinthians 6:14) can be so devastating to our prosperity.

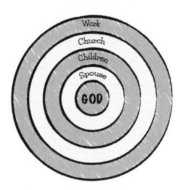

And the LORD *God formed man of the dust of the ground, and breathed into his nostrils the breath of life; and man became a living soul* (Genesis 2:7).

Thou shalt love the Lord thy God with all thy heart, and with all thy soul, and with all thy strength, and with all thy mind; and thy neighbor as thyself (Luke 10:27).

So God created man in his own image, in the image of God created he him; male and female created he them (Genesis 1:27).

God made us with multiple components. We were formed from the dust of the ground and will someday return to dust. Flesh, bone, and blood make up our physical beings. God also gave us a will and made us in His image, sovereign over our decisions. Each of us has a heart (inner being of who we really are), soul (life that extends past our days on this earth into eternity), strength (flesh), and mind (intellect). God also brought relationships into this discussion when He mentioned neighbors (others). The only way to love our neighbor as ourselves successfully is if we love ourselves. For one to love himself reflects an understanding that God made us in His image and that we are valuable, loved, and glorious. He makes everything glorious, and He made us! Understanding this concept helps us to love our Creator and to be satisfied with the way He made us. Balancing the multiple facets of who we are is critical for our wellness. We are spiritual beings, but we also are physical, emotional, and logical. True health and prosperity come from the balance of all aspects of who God made us to be.

The word "balance" is used eight times in the KJV, and we find the word "balances" ten times. We can also see the word "balance" in other versions, as follows.

1 occurrence – NKJV
3 occurrences – NIV
2 occurrences – NLT

And this the writing that was written, MENE, MENE, TEKEL, UPHARSIN. This is the interpretation of the thing: MENE;

God hath numbered thy kingdom, and finished it. TEKEL; Thou art weighed in the balances, and art found wanting. PERES; Thy kingdom is divided, and given to the Medes and Persians (Daniel 5:25-28).

A balance – a weighing device consisting of a rigid beam horizontally suspended by a low friction support at its center, with identical weight pans hung at either end. Place a known weight on one side and then put enough of a product on the other side to balance it. When level, the weights are equal. This represents one item opposed to the other.

The balanced life – a tool God can use. The key is not balancing family and work or family and God; it is having the proper focus. All components should work toward the same goal as we trust God truly in all we do.

At a leadership development seminar, I heard a speaker discuss motivational intelligence. We hear a lot about emotional intelligence, but I have not heard much in regard to motivational intelligence. This fascinating subject is one I plan to dig into further.

One of the examples in the presentation was of a child learning to walk. It has been estimated that a child learning to walk will fall an average of seventeen times per hour. Thank goodness for thick diapers, I guess! That is a lot of time on the ground. Based on this information, the attitude of children who refuse to give up is amazing. Their perseverance can last for days or even weeks while they attempt to conquer this milestone in their life. Without relying on excuses or fear of change, they display relentless persistence, unwavering confidence, infinite ability, and boundless self-motivation.

We all have that capability. The question is: Why do we stop trying so hard to accomplish a goal? If at one time we relentlessly pursued a goal without stopping because of a failure, why do we no longer have that persistence? We acted with perseverance initially because we had not yet learned that we should stop trying. As we get older we are taught to stop trying. It is really tragic that this is a reality, but it is.

Thomas Edison experimented with more than one thousand materials to invent the lightbulb. He was asked at one point, "How can you keep trying when you have failed so many times?" He replied that he did not fail; he learned what did not work. That is the attitude of a child.

Success is a by-product of goals and results. Goals and results are by-products of actions and skills. Actions and skills are by-products of thoughts and beliefs. We must alter our thoughts and beliefs before we can change the actions and skills, which will then lead to better goals and results that bring success.

The complete person can be understood by the complete athlete. A fifteen-year-old boy with a strong work ethic loved basketball. He was already 6'7" and was passionate about the game. Dominant in his league, he had parents committed to his success. He had everything he needed for success. He often practiced in the driveway for hours. A friend of the father visited and mentioned to the boy's father that he could really go far with a career in basketball. The father said, "He could, but he won't." The boy would practice only the aspects of the game he enjoyed. If he did not like something, he would not work on it. That was fine for the competition at fifteen years old when he was so much taller than everyone else, but when he got older and faced competition just as tall and more dedicated than he, his attitude would not get him to the next level. You see, he didn't have a complete game.

The principle fits in this section as well. A full life is about being balanced or complete. If you have no jump shot and work only on driving the lane, you will not be successful as the competition gets bigger and better. In like manner, if you do not take care of yourself physically and focus only on the spiritual, you may be too sick to minister at some point, but if you focus only on the physical and not the spiritual, you will forfeit your effectiveness in the kingdom of God. If you bank on playing basketball for a career and do not get an education, you may find yourself unemployed, without a back-up plan.

All of life requires us to be balanced. We need to possess the "complete" game. That is what this book is about—the "complete game," otherwise known as the balanced life.

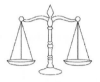

Chapter Two

Divine Healing

Healing signifies restoration to health or soundness; cure. It can also mean to ease or relieve in the case of emotional distress. God created the body to heal itself naturally. The human body is a self-healing organism. Our bodies are equipped to kill the cancer cells that we produce every day, fight infectious diseases, keep our arteries open, repair broken proteins, and combat the aging process.

God also designed stress, the "fight or flight" mechanism, for our benefit. When we find ourselves in a dangerous situation, the body releases cortisol that pumps us up and likely saves our lives. The problem is that our body functions as a self-healing organism only when we are not in the "fight or flight" mode. The constant stress we live in as part of today's society has a devastating effect on our health and well-being.

The Bible talks a lot about God's healing power. All the way back in Exodus 23:25 (NKJV), the Word says, "So you shall serve the LORD your God, and He will bless your bread and your water. And I will take sickness away from the midst of you." What an awesome verse not just about healing but about God's providing us with the food and water He has blessed, which will take sickness away! Proper nutrition is a key element to eliminating sickness. What is the balance between divine healing and healthy living? There are divine healing instances, but often healing is tied to our making the proper healthy choices.

Let's check out some passages of Scripture that deal with divine healing:

Who forgiveth all thine iniquities; who healeth all thy diseases (Psalm 103:3).

He sent his word, and healed them, and delivered them from their destructions (Psalm 107:20).

For I will restore health unto thee, and I will heal thee of thy wounds, saith the LORD; because they called thee an Outcast, saying, This is Zion, whom no man seeketh after (Jeremiah 30:17).

And Jesus went about all Galilee, teaching in their synagogues, and preaching the gospel of the kingdom, and healing all manner of sickness and all manner of disease among the people (Matthew 4:23).

Divine Healing

Heal the sick, cleanse the lepers, raise the dead, cast out devils: freely you have received, freely give (Matthew 10:8).

And Jesus went forth, and saw a great multitude, and was moved with compassion toward them, and he healed their sick (Matthew 14:14).

And these signs shall follow them that believe; In my name shall they cast out devils; . . . they shall lay hands on the sick, and they shall recover (Mark 16:17-18).

How God anointed Jesus of Nazareth with the Holy Ghost and with power; who went about doing good, and healing all that were oppressed of the devil; for God was with him (Acts 10:38).

God wants to heal our wounds, our diseases, and our sickness and deliver those who are oppressed of the devil. Sometimes He does that supernaturally, and sometimes He does it through nutrition and a healthy lifestyle.

I have heard numerous accounts of and even witnessed and experienced God's healing power. Some instances are amazing and supernatural. Some are small but faith-building nonetheless. As a child I joined the youth group at the church one Saturday morning. We had met at the church to load up for a canoeing trip. The orthodontist had adjusted my braces the day before, and I was in a lot of pain. This doesn't sound like a big deal, but to a young boy who had been longing for this canoeing trip, it was a huge disappointment. I couldn't enjoy it at all. Right before entering the van, I asked some of the elders to pray for me. We drove to the canoe livery, and as I loaded the canoe into the truck, I realized my mouth was not hurting at all. After all these years, I remember that small encounter with God's healing touch, and it still increases my faith. Usually I would have pain for three to five days after getting my braces adjusted, but this time the pain left within an hour of being prayed for. I had a great day canoeing!

In the church where I grew up, my family was one of the first to begin attending the church after it had been founded. One of the ladies in the church was diagnosed with brain cancer. The medical team had to do surgery, and when they removed the tumor, they removed the part of the brain that controlled her balance. They said she would never walk again. She was the grandmother of my best friend. During one service she asked her daughter to stand on the opposite side of the sanctuary. After her daughter walked to the other side of the sanctuary, she stood for the first time since the surgery and then walked across the front of the auditorium to her daughter. She pushed her wheelchair out of the church that day and left it at her doctor's office after her next appointment. The place erupted in praise when she got out of that wheelchair! The doctor had no explanation other than divine healing. She should never have been able to walk after that surgery, yet in an instant she was healed and spent many more years walking and praising God.

Divine Healing

I also recall a miracle for my best friend's younger sister. We hung out together all the time. When we were in our mid-teen years, she contracted an eye infection. Her eye was very swollen and red. Her parents brought her to the church and asked the elders to pray for her. One of our elders opened his eyes while praying, and he literally saw the redness and swelling disappear. I saw it from the viewpoint outside the office. When she went into the room for prayer, her eye was swollen and red, but when she came out a short while later, it was back to normal. The elder actually watched the swelling dissipate. It was a case of divine healing.

My biological grandfather passed away when I was very young. My grandmother remarried when I was still pretty young, and her husband became the grandfather I knew and spent time with while growing up. He was a good man but had never been in a church building. They were actually married in an event center instead of a church. He was a heavy smoker since his teens, and when I was still a child, he was diagnosed with emphysema and told if he didn't quit smoking he would be dead within a year. So he quit smoking but struggled with the effects of the disease for the rest of his life.

By the time I reached my late teens, his health started declining. He then got pneumonia; this coupled with the emphysema caused him to deteriorate rapidly. That was early 1993, and my fiancee and I planned to marry in June. My grandfather really wanted to live to see the wedding.

An evangelist had come to the church for a revival. On Sunday night the evangelist spoke a word of faith and told the congregation that if we knew of anyone who needed a healing, we needed to get that person to the service Monday night. My dad and I immediately thought of my grandfather. The next day my dad stopped by and told him what the evangelist had said. Although he had never been to church and wanted nothing to do with it, my grandfather agreed to attend that night.

Near the end of the service, the evangelist asked for anyone who needed a healing to come to stand in the front. This was a monumental task for my grandfather. He had been in the hospital the week before. Very weak, he couldn't walk far or stand long. He went up, and the evangelist went around the altar praying for people one at a time. For some reason he waited until almost last to pray for my grandfather. We were all shocked that he was able to stand so long and not fall over or come back to his seat. Eventually the evangelist reached him and said something in his ear. We still have no idea what was said. He then asked him to raise his hands; in a matter of a few seconds my grandfather received the Holy Ghost and was speaking in tongues. Miraculous, to say the least! Of course, we were ecstatic.

The next day he had to go back to the hospital. He was a different man, though. Although he was a good man, he was not a kind man. He was usually grumpy and could be rather difficult. He had some anger issues, but after receiving the Holy Ghost, he was kind and gentle, a quite different person. After a week in the hospital, he got out and came home. We had talked to him about baptism. We didn't understand why he didn't get a physical healing, but we knew he needed to be baptized.

On a Monday night, the doctors wanted him to be admitted to the hospital again. He asked if we would baptize him before he checked into the hospital. We had a family baptismal service that night. We expected him to come out of the water healed from the emphysema and pneumonia. He was spiritually healed and God delivered him from many emotional wounds, but physically he still had to go to the hospital. The sting of death was gone, and a few days later he passed away, a couple of weeks before our wedding.

My best friend's grandmother got out of a wheelchair and walked out of church pushing her wheelchair. My grandfather came to the altar for healing and was forever changed but died a few weeks later. Why did God heal one and not the other? I have witnessed many incidences of divine healing. I have seen people delivered, but my grandfather died.

This is not a book on the gifts of the Spirit, but I do feel the need to discuss them briefly here. Divine healing meshes with the gifts of healing mentioned by Paul to the Corinthians. "To another faith by the same Spirit; to another the gifts of healing by the same Spirit" (1 Corinthians 12:9).

One of the gifts of the Spirit is the "gifts of healing." The Bible does not say the "gift" of healing but the "gifts" of healing. It is not a gift that someone possesses so that he can heal anyone at any time. If so, he would have a line at his door that would never end. We do see in the New Testament account after account of divine healing. I believe that "gifts of healing" operate in three primary areas: physical (cancer, diseases, for example), mental (depression, nervous disorders, and so on), and spiritual (demonic spirits, deliverance). Many times in Jesus' ministry, spirits were cast out and healing followed. Eternity consists of the past, the present, and the future. We live in the present, but God lives in all three. Thus, He can take something and restore it to a former state. Jesus can connect the past to the present.

He can also connect the future to the present. In Matthew 12:10-13 the Bible tells us of a man who "had his hand withered. . . . Then saith he to the man, Stretch forth thine hand. And he stretched it forth; and it was restored whole, like as the other." A broken hand may take six weeks to heal, but it will heal over time if it is set properly. Jesus can make that six weeks happen right now. He is not confined to time. That is the divine aspect of healing when He takes what once was or what will be and makes it the present reality.

Sometimes He chooses to heal in a divine fashion, sometimes He heals by our bodies' natural healing process, and sometimes He chooses not to heal physically at all. Often, though, we have a lot to do with it. Divine healing is at times a measure of our faith. But natural healing is the subject we will now address.

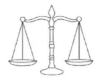

Chapter Three

Natural Healing

Dr. Andrew Wiel is known for his holistic health approach. He graduated from Harvard with a doctorate degree. In his video, *Spontaneous Healing*, he discusses the primary reasons he didn't want to practice medicine:

1) Standard practice did not take an approach to health that should be a doctor's focus.
2) He wouldn't want that done to him.

He spent the next ten years traveling the world and studying different methods of medical practices. He is also a botanist. He studied plants and herbs while believing in a certain aspect of the divine. He also stresses the importance of surrounding yourself with those who believe in healing. Healing is the norm, not the exception. God designed the human body to heal itself.

Both divine healing and natural healing are part of God's overall plan. God provided diet restrictions in the

Old Testament. Sickness and healing are facets of our lives. We have seen and experienced them. Yet we experience thorns that are necessary for us to grow up and grow strong. We will discuss thorns in more detail later.

My father goes to a doctor who is a genius. He graduated from medical school far ahead of schedule and started his own practice. When my dad asked him about nutrition and how it could aid in the resolution of some medical problems, the doctor's answer was shocking. He said he didn't know anything about nutrition. A somewhat recent graduate with a doctorate degree admitted that through all that schooling they had not taught anything about nutrition. He was very educated on different chemicals and drugs and how they react to our bodies but was never instructed how our diet can be the cause of—and sometimes the answer to—our health issues.

> *Then God said, "Let the land produce vegetation: seed-bearing plants and trees on the land that bear fruit with seed in it, according to their various kinds." And it was so. The land produced vegetation: plants bearing seed according to their kinds and trees bearing fruit with seed in it according to their kinds. And God saw that it was good* (Genesis 1:11-12, NIV).

God set principles, standards, and laws when He created the earth and humanity. You have to learn to work with these creative laws and principles. You can try to ignore them, but they will break you if you do not recognize them. For example, gravity is one of the laws established in creation. You can stand on the roof of a building and scream, "I don't believe in gravity," while jumping off the building. Regardless of whether or not you believe in gravity, you will feel the effects of gravity when you hit the concrete sidewalk.

You can eat an apple and plant the core with the seeds in it. You can say that you want to grow an orange, you can put a picture of an orange on the ground beside the spot where you planted the apple seed, and you can even pour out an orange-juice offering. But you planted an apple seed, and if the conditions are right an apple tree will begin to sprout from the ground. That is a principle of creation. Things reproduce according to their kinds. We can call this the law of sowing and reaping. If you plant apples, you will grow apples. This is a principle that stretches beyond horticulture. It pertains to all areas of our lives.

My high school drafting teacher has been a highly influential person in my life. He taught us that everyone has to pay his dues sometime in life. Shortly before my class graduated, he told us we could choose to pay our dues immediately by attending college and working hard. Later in life, we would reap the benefits of a good job and a better working environment. Or we could get a job at once and live an easier life than the friends who went to college and invested in their futures. Then, we would pay our dues later when we were stuck in dead-end jobs, watching our friends move ahead in their careers.

Sowing and reaping is a powerful principle that God instituted. It also has a powerful relationship to health and wellness. I recently saw a breakdown of our health makeup and what contributes to it. The chart showed the following breakdown.

20 percent of health is DNA
30 percent of health is behaviors
10 percent is physical environment
40 percent is socioeconomic factors
(education, job, income, etc.)

However accurate this chart is, I hear a common reason for health issues: "It is in my DNA to be overweight," or "I have an uphill road because of my genes or family history." I have always believed that most of the family history is more a history of habits than a story of DNA. Most people eat the same foods at the same times and have the same lifestyle as their families. So if your standard evening as a child consisted of eating large helpings of fried food, always having a sweet dessert, and then sitting to watch something for a few hours before eating a high-calorie snack before bed, that may be the driver to your health status. On the contrary, if you grew up eating a meal with veggies and fruits, not having dessert or late-night meals, but you typically took a walk or engaged in other physical activity in the evenings, that may be the driver to your health status.

According to this list, 30 percent of health is behaviors, and only 20 percent of your health is DNA. Even if you have a challenging family history, you can change your behaviors; in other terms, start to "sow" different seeds to make an impact on your health.

The other large percentage is the socioeconomic factor. I conclude that most of the socioeconomic factors are powerful and influential because they affect your behaviors. Your job can affect your health, but you can overcome some of that by your behaviors. For example, it is common for welders to smoke. Welding creates a smoke the welder will inhale, but more and better safety devices are coming out to limit the ingestion of smoke when welding. That factor will affect your health. If you choose to smoke a cigarette because all your co-workers are smoking during break, you create a behavior that can be avoided. So I would argue that some of the socio-economic factors are really behaviors as well.

Either way, DNA is a factor in our health but not the largest factor. It can be overcome. It is very important to accept this and not submit yourself to the belief that your DNA predestines you to an unhealthy life. That is a lie from the enemy whose desire is to kill, to steal, and to destroy. Realize that even if you have a challenging family history, you can change your behaviors and lead a healthier life. It is certainly worth a try!

These are all principles God ordained when He created the world. We reap what we sow. This principle reaches into every area of our lives. It is also important to note that you reap more than you sow. One kernel of corn can produce a stalk with two to four ears. Each ear of corn has approximately eight hundred kernels of corn. So one kernel can generate between 1600 and 3200 more kernels of corn. If you were to take an average of 2400 and plant all of those the next year, your one kernel could yield 5,760,000 kernels in just two seasons.

You always reap more than you sow. That is part of the law of sowing and reaping. Our actions and decisions have a lasting impact on our life.

Chapter Four

Healthy Living

One of my favorite sayings is: "Common sense is no longer common—it should be called uncommon sense." The diet restrictions in the Old Testament give us some guidelines that make sense. What can we do to avoid some of the horrific diseases that plague Christians and non-Christians alike these days? There is hardly anyone who has not been affected either personally or through someone he or she loves by heart disease, cancer, a stroke, or diabetes. Most diseases that ravage America today can be prevented or controlled through proper nutrition, herbs, and weight control.

When I was a pastor, I visited an elderly couple in our church who could no longer attend services due to health issues. We had a nice visit, and the wife actually presented me with some desires for her funeral service, knowing she would not be around much longer. They were some of the sweetest people, and I truly loved them as their pastor. She had a stroke that left her partially paralyzed and unable to get around well. One of her base issues was diabetes. Most of her other problems were magnified due to the diabetes.

She said, "Pastor Shaun, the doctor told me years ago, when I was first diagnosed with pre-diabetes, that if I lost ten pounds I would never have to worry about diabetes or any of the complications that come with it. I never lost those ten pounds, though, so I'll never know."

A measly ten pounds would have given her a much better, longer life and probably would have prevented the stroke that sent her to a premature grave.

One day at work during a break, I went into the kitchen to grab my lunch. A co-worker was eating a huge cheeseburger with bacon, mayo, and all the "fixin's" on it, along with a side of fries.

He saw my rather healthy lunch and commented, "I know that I won't live as long as you healthy people, but I am sure going to die happy eating stuff I enjoy."

After thinking about it, I realized he probably will not die happy. After the effects of his eating and lack of exercise catch up with him, he will battle with the products of his lifestyle and likely not be active or enjoy the hobbies he loves, such as fishing, hunting, and spending time with his family. He struggles to walk due to his weight, and he is still fairly young. He may be happy when he takes a bite of that burger, but in the long run, he will struggle due to his unhealthy lifestyle. It is actually sad. Pay your dues now or pay them later.

While writing this book, I had to make some adjustments. My family history is not very good. My father and his mother both had diabetes. His father died of a heart attack in his fifties, and he also lost an uncle in his fifties from a heart attack. I have worked hard to maintain my weight and try to live a healthy life. I am as busy as anyone. We are very involved in church and with our children. I coached or helped coach baseball and football teams and have been a Bible quizzing coach for many years, which are all demanding on my time. I am also an executive of a growing company that keeps me extremely busy. I try to run a minimum of three or four times a week and do moderate weightlifting and sit-ups. I have run a few half-marathons and run 5Ks regularly.

During the writing of this book, our family spent a month in Ohio, where I worked at the corporate office. It was a great time! The company put us in a cabin on eighty-two acres with a pond and all kinds of fun things to do. It is a long drive from Texas to Ohio, and while in Ohio I was out of my routine. I didn't eat well, I rarely got my workout time in, and I stayed up late visiting with family. At the end of the month, I was scheduled to have my wellness exam that allows us to earn credits toward our health insurance premiums. This can be a significant saving if I earn the credits.

For the first time, I was borderline for a couple of the tests. I was close to pre-diabetes. This was a wake-up call. I have always lived by the thought that "the exceptions aren't what kills you; it is the rule that kills you." If you eat well and work out regularly, it doesn't hurt you to miss a day or be a little careless with your eating occasionally. The older I get, the harder it is to cheat and not feel the effect. I usually considered traveling as a "cheat" time, but I didn't normally travel for a month at a time.

Putting those scenarios together at the same time caused my blood work to come back worse than it had in years.

You see, when I got married, I was very thin and didn't eat healthy at all. I had no worries about weight or health. Then as we started having children and I started pastoring, I started to gain weight. I reached 199 pounds, about 70 pounds heavier than my weight when I married. No longer healthy, I needed to be concerned about my weight. I started walking. Gradually, that turned into running a little bit, and then a friend at work talked me into running a Memorial Day 5K with him. At that point I was hooked. I was still as busy as before, but I made an early morning workout a priority. "Bodily exercise profiteth little," but it does profit as long as you keep it in perspective and balance.

Solomon opened the Book of Proverbs by telling us the purpose of the book.

> *Their* [the proverbs'] *purpose is to teach people wisdom and discipline, and to help them understand the insights of the wise. Their purpose is to teach people to live disciplined and successful lives, to help them do what is right, just, and fair. These proverbs will give insight to the simple, knowledge and discernment to the young. Let the wise listen to these proverbs and become even wiser. Let those with understanding receive guidance by exploring the meaning in these proverbs and parables, the words of the wise and their riddles.*

Fear of the LORD is the foundation of true knowledge, but fools despise wisdom and discipline (Proverbs 1:2-7, NLT).

As the wise Solomon stated, the purpose of the book is to teach people wisdom and discipline. The two go hand in hand. If we can apply the wisdom of Proverbs, we will receive instruction in discipline and get wiser. The basis for the entire book is remembering that the fear of the Lord is the beginning, the foundation, of all wisdom. No matter how wise we get, we can never get above that.

Wisdom tells us that the only way to get it is to value it and search for it. Read, study, communicate with God—that is the route to get wise. This comes only when coupled with discipline. Discipline is also critical in the natural sense. We often discuss the importance of the spiritual disciplines of prayer, fasting, and study of the Word but neglect the discipline in our bodies that will allow us to be more productive in our spiritual walk. As the wise Solomon also said:

> *Do not mix with winebibbers, Or with glut-tonous eaters of meat; For the drunkard and the glutton will come to poverty, And drowsiness will clothe a man with rags* (Proverbs 23:20-21, NKJV).

The problem of neglect of our bodies seems to be especially bad with those in the ministry. We can be spiritual yet unbalanced. We don't do the kingdom of God any good dead. We must take care of our bodies. We get into the habits of eating late, consuming junk food, taking advantage of clergy parking spots and elevators, and spending too much time sitting. These all take a terrible toll on our bodies. We all get so busy that fast food is the easiest choice, and we try to justify eating after service because Jesus and the apostles did so.

But as Eric Schlosser says, "Fast food is popular because it's convenient, it's cheap, and it tastes good. But the real cost of eating fast food never appears on the menu." If you came up with the worst possible food as far as nutrition goes, you probably couldn't come up with something worse than fast food.

Many have used the verse of Scripture that states, "But reject profane and old wives' fables, and exercise yourself toward godliness. For bodily exercise profits a little, but godliness is profitable for all things, having promise of the life that now is and of that which is to come" (1 Timothy 4:7-8, NKJV).

Our major pursuit must be godliness. Godliness is not just for this life but for the next life as well. We need to realize two things, though: 1) we live in a much different society than they lived in Jesus' days, and 2) the Scripture doesn't tell us that bodily exercise is unprofitable but that it profits little in the realm of eternity. In biblical times people walked almost everywhere. They constantly exerted themselves while traveling, whether walking, sailing, or even riding. They ate natural foods that weren't genetically engineered, and they didn't have a clue of some of the fats and processed foods we put in our bodies. They ate fish, olive oil, honey, and bread with unbleached, whole grains but no pork or bottom-feeding fish. They didn't avoid meat, but they were balanced and did not have to worry about synthetic food filled with preservatives. They had plenty of physical activity as part of their everyday life.

We don't have to worry about excessive physical exercise nearly as much as we must worry about avoiding disease and the premature breakdown of our bodies. First Thessalonians 5:23 states (NKJV, my emphases), "Now may the God of peace Himself sanctify you completely; and *may your whole* spirit, soul, *and body be preserved blameless* at the coming of our Lord Jesus Christ."

According to Genesis 2:7 (NKJV), "The LORD God formed man of the dust of the ground, and breathed into his nostrils the breath of life; and man became a living being." Man became a body (formed of the dust of the ground), a soul (given the breath of life), and a spiritual being (made in the image of God). It is critically important to view the entirety of our being when we consider the balance. In that case, we must look at health.

It only makes sense that God created the body to heal itself, and instead of just looking for drugs from medical science to counteract symptoms, we should look toward giving our bodies the proper nutrition to keep problems from happening. So much of what we get from restaurants, grocery stores, and especially fast food locations has little to no nutritional value. Whether it is genetically engineered to the point that our body can't use it or just cooked in such a way that kills all the nutrients, some of it may end up hurting us more than helping us.

As we enter this section of the book, I would like to recommend a few books as supplements to this book.

You should not just read them but buy them so you can keep them as reference works. This is just like budgeting or any other area of your life that requires discipline. You have to keep it in front of you, or you will slip away from it. I don't agree with everything in any of these books, but there the power of the balance comes in. Read, take notes, and glean from what you learn. Throw away what doesn't work, and hold fast to that which is good. As I mentioned previously, I truly believe that the exceptions will not kill you if they are truly exceptions. What really matters is what you do consistently—day in and day out, with an exception only a few times throughout the year.

I despise dieting books. It is amazing that a "new" diet concept comes out every year: the Atkins diet, the grapefruit diet, the no carb, the cabbage soup diet, the flat belly diet, eating according to your blood type, the Keto diet, and the "you fill in the blank" diet. Diet books are ever on the best-seller list, yet the simplest concepts are the most difficult things to do.

A few of the things that will transform your life the most fall into the category of things that are simple yet extremely difficult, such as managing your finances. Financial stress is the number one cause of divorce in America, yet we all know that all we need to do is spend less than we make. So simple and so difficult. Saying no to spending is extremely difficult. If it wasn't, no one would be broke and stressed out over his finances. We want to eat out, drive a nice car, and live in a nice house, but the result is stress and more bills than we can afford to pay. We know that daily prayer and Bible reading are the foundation for victorious living as a Christian. Yet it is difficult to discipline our mind and take time to pray every day. Simple but difficult.

Dieting and food. We need to eat. Eating too little will kill you. Eating too much will kill you. The key is to eat what you need in order to be healthy and productive. Eat fewer calories and burn more calories. That is simple to understand yet hard to do. Dieting books come along, sell numerous copies, and give people hope that this will be the solution to their struggle with their weight. Still, all they do is perpetuate the endless cycle of losing and gaining weight. The key is a balanced and healthy life-style. Constantly cycling through weight gain and loss is unhealthy in and of itself.

As a child, I was an unwilling participant in various dieting fads. I ate alfalfa sprouts on everything for weeks. There is nothing wrong with alfalfa sprouts, but the problem with a diet such as that is one gets tired of eating the same thing all the time. I remember eating cabbage soup for multiple meals. That stuff was horrible on the stomach. I didn't even need to lose weight. We did no carb, low carb, blood type, and cyclical eating. We lost a lot of weight and gained it all back.

My metabolism allowed me to eat anything and sometimes everything in my youth. Even in college I would take four peanut butter and jelly sandwiches, a bag of chips, a box of Little Debbie snack cakes (yes, a box), and a half-gallon of water for lunch. I would eat a couple of double cheeseburgers from McDonald's on my way home to hold me over until dinner. I rebelled against diets as we had gone through the newest book and diet fad of the day repeatedly.

After growing up and getting married, I gradually put on weight. I seemed to gain weight with each of my wife's pregnancies, but she would lose it and I didn't. One day I realized I had to stop. My wife had always been very health-conscious, but I didn't follow. So we started working together on being healthier. I want to expose you to some of the most impacting and helpful books we experienced that helped us on our journey.

God's Way for Healthy Living

My wife and I have read a lot of books on health and nutrition. The volume about healthy living I consider the most beneficial is *Greater Health God's Way* by Stormie Omartian. Of all the health and diet books to which I have been exposed, hers addresses the power of a balanced and healthy life better than any other.

She dissects health into seven essential categories that we need to cultivate so we can live as productive and healthy as God desires us to live. The seven steps are:

1) Peaceful living
2) Pure food
3) Proper exercise
4) Plenty of water
5) Prayer and fasting
6) Fresh air and sunshine
7) Perfect rest

Bodily exercise profits little, but a well-balanced, healthy lifestyle profits a lot. If more of God's people lived according to this, the kingdom of God would profit immeasurably. Each of these steps is something we have applied to our lives and try to apply each and every day. I want to touch on each of the major topics and put some of my thoughts and lifestyle adjustments with them.

Peaceful Living

Stress is a part of life. How we react to events can impact our health. Often many little things lead to major stress rather than just one big event. Prayer and Bible reading are great ways to prepare your heart and mind for a day. I want to put a plug in here for morning prayer and state how important it is to start your day by spending time with God. There is no replacement for asking God to help you through your day before you begin the day.

Another key is that exercise helps you deal with stress. Healthy eating reduces the stress on your immune system and body in general.

Stormie talks about the importance of simplifying our life. I believe that two of the greatest ways to avoid stress are by having healthy relationships and staying out of debt. I will talk more about finances later in this book, but financial pressure is the number one cause of divorce in the US. Debt creates a lot of stress on a marriage and in our lives. Peaceful living is critical if we are going to live a victorious life and give our best to God.

I work for a metal manufacturing facility. A guy who ran a press told me I didn't understand how stressful it was running that press. He had spent over forty years running that press. He would push two buttons, slide the bar into the press, and push the button. I thought it was interesting that although he didn't manage people, didn't deal with a lot of high-cost material, and didn't have to handle any work issues at home, he was stressed. To someone who has a lot of responsibility, it could sound ridiculous that this guy was stressed by sliding a bar in and hitting a button. But to this guy it was stressful.

God designed each of us with different stress and tolerance levels. It is important to understand what your stress level is and what you can take, then operate within that level. God won't give us more than we can bear, but we need to avoid taking on more than we should bear. More on that later.

Pure Food

We try to operate in a "way of life for eating, not a diet. . . . It is the way to eat whether you need to lose weight, gain weight, stay the same, or get well. It is totally satisfying, and you do not have hunger as a way of life. To sum it up in a nutshell it is: *Eating pure food the way that God made it,* or as close as possible to the way He made it" (p. 52, my emphasis).

For example, my wife and I don't concentrate on the fat content or fixate on the calorie count. We focus more on which foods to avoid and to include, such as the reasons we need to include whole grains and avoid white flour and white rice. What we eat has a tremendous impact on our feelings, energy level, weight, and health.

We have 260 trainable tastebuds. You can train your body to like certain foods, and the more you eat good foods, the better they will taste. The more you eat processed foods, the more you crave them. Processed foods are also very low in nutritional value. That leaves you hungrier sooner because the food didn't fulfill your nutritional needs. So if you train your body to like carrots or almonds as your go-to snack, you will get more nutritional value and consume something much better for you. This is an extremely important part of healthy living.

Proper Exercise

Exercise is critical if we want to live healthy and happy lives. Numerous studies and resources support the value of exercise. I would also like to mention another book, *Younger Next Year*, written by an overweight and overstressed lawyer from New York City and a doctor who worked with him to get healthy. The doctor is an evolutionist—I wholly disagree with him in this regard—but he goes through a number of things that helped the lawyer get "younger" in his health and well-being by exercising and living a healthier lifestyle. Once again, take the good from the book and leave the bad. I found it to be a motivating read. It is critical to read books on healthy living and re-read the best ones. They help you keep things in perspective and motivate you to live a healthy lifestyle.

I am an advocate for living an active lifestyle. It is more of an attitude than a specific rule. I rarely took advantage of clergy parking spots. I would always try to park at the far end of the lot and walk. I felt that was another way to get in a few extra steps. I try to use the stairs instead of the elevator as much as possible. Even when on an upper floor, you can plan a little extra time and use the stairs when you have the opportunity. We can't stop the aging process, but we can slow it. Thinking actively and trying to take advantage of opportunities to involve a few more steps add up in the long run. This is not a substitute for having a regular exercise routine as part of your week, but it does help.

When I was a kid, I was a "thumb drummer," constantly playing the drums with my thumbs and fingers at a table—or anywhere else, for that matter. I struggled to sit still and probably would have been on medication if I was in today's school system. This constant drumming drove my dad nuts. He would frequently put his hand on mine to stop my incessant drumming. I later learned from an article that thumb drumming, hair twirling, and other nervous-habit type activities can add up to burning over a hundred calories a day. I don't advocate driving people nuts by drumming, but espouse thinking and living actively. Instead of taking a nap when you have an extra hour, go for a bike ride or take a walk. Instead of golfing with a cart, walk. Take up Frisbee golf or something that isn't strenuous but keeps you active.

Plenty of Water

A huge percent of our body is comprised of water. I have seen a variety of numbers expressing the percentage of the body that is water. Some estimate that as much as 85 percent of the human body is water. The body is constantly losing water through the ordinary processes of life. Water is extremely critical to many bodily functions and is a transporter of nutrients through the body. I have read many accounts that recommend we drink sixty-four ounces of water a day. The amount needed varies widely, based on a person's size and level of activity.

Some people suggest not drinking while eating (or shortly before or after a meal), but I do not agree. I have to drink while eating, or I do not feel well. My wife, on the other hand, cannot drink while eating, or she does not feel well. I believe everyone is different. I have asked doctors about this, and their opinions vary as well. One doctor said he believes it is very important to drink while eating because it helps to get the digestive process working. Others say it dilutes the digestive juices. Since God made us individuals, I believe the key is to drink plenty of water all day long. Drink during a meal if it works for you, and don't drink during a meal if it doesn't work for you. Probably as important as drinking water is what you do not drink.

Moderation is a key. Some people don't like coffee but like the smell of it; my wife is one of those. Fortunately, I like neither its smell nor its taste. Many beverages common today are so full of calories, sugar, and other bad ingredients that people don't even realize how many calories they consume while drinking. Eliminating high-calorie drinks can solve a lot of financial problems and cut a lot of calories.

At one point I totally stopped drinking soda and lost ten pounds in a few weeks. Most people don't realize how many calories they consume when they drink a soda or a latte. You have to walk approximately thirty minutes to offset one can of Coke. If you are drinking a couple of cans a day, it takes a lot of walking just to cover those empty calories.

Another important factor is pure water. Depending on where you live, tap water may not be your optimal choice, and having a water system to cleanse the water in your home can be a very worthwhile investment. Drink lots of pure water, and it will make a huge difference in your well-being.

Prayer and Fasting

Spiritual peace is a vital part of serene living. Many of our troubles can be washed away by spending time in prayer and the Word of God. I am a straightforward person and not emotionally connected. I have to put effort into considering "feelings." I have purposely read the Book of Psalms with the purpose of paying attention to the emotions David expressed. He had incredible lows and highs emotionally. His writings reflect these ups and downs. Job also experienced incredible highs and deep lows while going through his trial. It is not something I relate to easily, but I have endeavored to understand this dynamic with which many people deal. Reading Job and the Psalms has helped me see more clearly the calming effect that the Word can introduce into someone's life.

Prayer, the Word, and fasting are critical disciplines that bring peace to our lives. They help us get other things out of the way and connect to God. I have gone through phases of frequent meal fasts. I have also had times of little fasting of meals but intentional withdrawal from media and other distractions. These help us find a balanced, healthy lifestyle in a very chaotic world.

Stormie has some great lists on what to do and what not to do during a fast and some excellent guidelines in regard to fasting. Numerous other writings on the subject of fasting are excellent resources as well. Joy Haney has written some excellent books on prayer and fasting that I highly recommend.

Fresh Air and Sunshine

Too many people go to work in the dark, work in an office or factory all day, and then go home to sit in front of a computer or TV until they go to bed. They include no activity, no motion, and no sunshine all day and get up the next day to repeat the process. This is both unnatural and unhealthy.

One year for my birthday my wife asked me to plan an ideal day, and she would make it happen. After some thought, I made my decision. At that time we were living in Ohio, and we used wood for our primary heat source. I loved going into the forest to chop and split logs, so I chose to get up early and chop wood all day with the kids. Then I had a date with my wife for dinner. Most people think it is crazy to consider that an ideal day, but I loved having quality time with my wife and kids and spending the entire day in the fresh air and sunshine. Now in my mid-forties, I work in an office, but I am outside as much as possible.

Even when I lived in the Houston area in summer, you typically found me outside on a day off: getting up early for a morning run or bike ride, working in the yard, playing basketball with my kids and their friends, coaching one of my kids' teams, or taking the kids to the park for a round of disc golf. Fresh air and sunshine are refreshing and invigorating. Our tastebuds get used to the food choices we make. I used to love Coke and sweet tea. Now I can hardly stand to drink sweet tea and love plain, unsweet tea, which is much healthier. Success breeds success. In the same way, being outside and active makes you want to be outside and active more often.

When I fail to run, bike, or lift weights too long, I struggle to get back into the habit. I have to retrain my muscles. In February 2014 I ran a half-marathon, finishing in under two hours, which was my goal. I was in pretty good shape. Due to extenuating circumstances, my workout routine dropped off for almost a year. One of our children was hospitalized for six months, many of those months in a hospital more than four hours from our home. Lots of late-night drives and the need to keep up with work, family, and a sick kid took a toll on my workout routine and eating habits. It was very hard to get back into it. What was half-marathon shape turned into a struggle to run a 5K. But just as when I started running, I had to get up and put one foot in front of the other and make it happen. Those runs were painfully slow, and sometimes a mile was all I would get in. It was much easier to get back into running shape once I got going, but it was very difficult to get up early and get started. Once again, success breeds success.

Get up, get outside, and enjoy life. Fresh air and sunshine are healthy and a necessary part of your lifestyle. Hunting, fishing, gardening, golf, going to the park, playing a sport, or taking a walk are all excellent activities for a healthy lifestyle. As Nike advertised in the '90s—just do it!

Perfect Rest

Sleep is a huge subject. Machines, sleep clinics, sleep tests, and narcotics are all common subjects related to sleep. People go to great lengths to get rest. Everyone longs for good sleep. One of the most common questions in the morning is "Did you sleep well?" One thing is certain: sleep is essential to good health. When you sleep well, you feel better, and it makes exercise, prayer, and Bible reading much easier.

Sleep is an area I really struggle in. I can usually fall asleep really quickly and sleep hard, but I don't sleep long. I am writing this section on a plane. I went to bed about 11 PM and had to get up at 3 AM to catch my flight. I am wired to awake before my alarm regardless of what time I set it, and I woke up this morning at 2:30. Almost everyone on the flight is sleeping, but I am writing. Even though I have gone for extended periods of time averaging four hours of sleep per night, I try not to put myself in the position for that to be the norm any more. I have realized the importance of rest. I work hard on getting to bed earlier. I try to make sure that I get real rest and more of it. If I am going to wake up early, I need to get to bed early. As the old saying goes, "Early to bed and early to rise makes a man healthy, wealthy, and wise." I am not sure how well it has worked, but I will keep trying.

I have learned that when you are balanced, living in peace, eating good food, exercising, drinking plenty of good water, praying and fasting (feeding your spiritual person), and getting fresh air and sunshine, good sleep will be a byproduct. I remember how well I have slept on trips where I spent a lot of time in the outdoors, ate well, worked hard, and removed myself from the stress of daily life. That is a good example of the steps coming together and producing perfect rest.

There are such things as "sleep stealers," and noting some of these is important. Overeating and eating toxin-forming foods can be sleep stealers. I have heard people joke about "pizza dreams" or jokingly question whether a dream was from God or from too much greasy food the night before. The truth is, what we eat does affect how we sleep.

Another huge aspect is a negative state of mind—worry, fear, and mental anxiety. Paul wrote in 2 Timothy 1:7 (NLT) that "God has not given us a spirit of fear and timidity, but of power, love, and self-discipline." The self-discipline to which this verse refers is disciplined thoughts. Either fear and worry will control us, or faith will overcome the fear and worry the world constantly puts in front of us. This is a large factor in today's world. Negative media bombards us twenty-four hours a day. When you go to a restaurant they have the news on; when you go to the dentist or doctor the news is on in the lobby. It seems impossible to get away from the barrage of negativity. The Constant Negative Network, otherwise known as CNN, dominates our lives. Bombings, shootings, viruses, disease, war, famine, earthquakes, and all-out disaster are thrown in our faces constantly. It almost sounds like Matthew 24!

I mentioned earlier that in the Psalms David addressed many emotions that we deal with and exposed his ups and downs better than any other author in the Scripture. He was scared, depressed, distracted, angry, joyous, victorious, and excited, and he shared that in the Bible. He opened up and displayed his deepest fears. In Psalm 118:6 (NIV) David said, "The LORD is with me; I will not be afraid. What can mere mortals do to me?" He probably slept well that night. Even if Saul was hunting David like a wild animal, even when he was hiding in a cave with a bunch of misfits and rejects, even if he was being sought by the Philistines, he could step away from it all and say, "Because God is with me, I don't have anything to worry about."

David started Psalm 27 thus:

The LORD is my light and my salvation; whom shall I fear? The LORD is the strength of my life; of whom shall I be afraid? When the wicked, even mine enemies and my foes, came upon me to eat up my flesh, they stumbled and fell.

This entire chapter is a powerful way to help us deal with fear and torment. Learning to trust God regardless of our circumstances brings peace that passes all understanding.

Sleeping too much is a problem as well. Some people sleep too much, and their level of mental activity is far more than their level of physical activity. It is just being out of balance. I interview a lot of people. People who really know themselves know that their weakness is their strength taken to the extreme. For example, if I ask someone his greatest strength and he tells me it is his attention to detail, that person probably struggles to see the big picture. If he really knows himself, he knows he is great at handling details. But not many detail people are big vision people, and they know it. Sleep is needed, but too much can be a negative.

Some success factors for sleeping well include getting to bed early. I know that when we don't go to bed early or make that a priority, it destroys the next day. I feel good when I get to bed early and get up in time to pray, read, exercise, and eat breakfast before work. Then at the end of that day I am ready for bed, and if I make going to bed early a priority, I usually fall asleep quickly and sleep well. So it repeats itself. Remember the cycle to success and the forming of a habit pay great dividends in life. I tell our kids on Saturday nights that the battle in Sunday morning worship service is usually won by getting to bed at a decent hour on Saturday night and guarding what you see and listen to on Saturday nights. It does make a difference.

My wife and I grew up in polar opposite homes when it comes to bed. My dad worked an early morning shift, and our house was silent and dark early. This was not the case in my wife's home as she grew up. So when we married, we had to compromise, and she usually turns something on quietly in the background and we have a dark room. When it is not dark I struggle to sleep long. I can fall asleep quickly but don't sleep as well if it is not dark and fairly quiet. We have some friends who take a box fan with them when they travel because they need the noise to sleep. Whatever works for you, know it and be disciplined to stick to it. Taking a few minutes to unwind and "unscreen" before bed is important. I have read studies that talk about the engagement our brains have when we look at a screen (TV, iPad, phone, etc.), and it can hinder your sleep.

Stay away from caffeine in the evening. Some people say it doesn't bother them, but I am sure it doesn't help either! These are important steps to good rest.

Putting It All Together

I have spent this much time and space on these topics because they comprise a balanced approach to healthy living, not a fad diet. It addresses a disciplined lifestyle, which is really the answer to healthy living. In the last chapter of her book, Stormie says, "Always keep in mind there is a fine line between grace (God does it) and obedience (I do my part). Doing it all by yourself is impossible. And if you cry, 'Grace!' over your sick, overweight body and then go have a chocolate doughnut and a soda, that won't work either. There needs to be a balance." Ask God for help, and then do your part.

I often said when I was pastoring that our level of obedience needs to match our level of knowledge. We have access to a tremendous amount of knowledge. We can research all kinds of facts, we hear amazing messages from the Word of God (available online now at any time of the day or night), and we have the Bible on our phones. We have so much knowledge at our fingertips it is mind-boggling. Yet frequently we do not match our obedience with the knowledge we have. We have to raise our level of obedience to our level of knowledge. Then we get more revelation and insight. We are constantly being fed, but if we don't raise our level of obedience, we are no more than gluttons.

The Dead Sea is the lowest point on earth's dry land. Nothing can live there. Even people who cannot swim can swim in the Dead Sea because it is impossible to sink due to the high salt content. It has inlets for water to flow into it but no outlet. Taking in and never giving or constantly learning and never obeying lead to death in the spiritual, physical, and all other areas of our life.

I love that God specializes in making things new. The Bible opens with the amazing story of Creation. God made something from nothing and then made something beautiful out of a mess. He can do that with us. He actually makes it a habit to take the mess we have made of our lives and make something brand-new out of it.

> *Therefore if any man be in Christ, he is a new creature: old things are passed away; behold, all things are become new* (2 Corinthians 5:17).

I love this verse. When I mess things up, I can trust that since I am in Christ, I can be made new again.

I also love David's prayer after his sin with Bathsheba. He began this section by asking God to make a clean heart in him.

*Create in me a clean heart, O God; and
renew a right spirit within me. Cast me not
away from thy presence; and take not thy
holy spirit from me. Restore unto me the
joy of thy salvation; and uphold me with
thy free spirit* (Psalm 51:10-12).

That is one of the most amazing attributes of God. He is a creator.

I work for a metal bar grating manufacturer. We take raw material such as coils of steel and wire and turn it into grating. We also fabricate. Fabricating is taking the manufactured product and adapting it for its final use. So we can buy coils of steel, slit them into slit coil, un-coil them into bar, weld them into grating, and then take that manufactured product and cut it and weld on it so it can be installed into a finished application. I find it fascinating to manufacture something every day.

When I started at this company, we did not manufacture many of our products. We did manufacture a few products, but most of the time we bought grating and just fabricated it. Through the years we vertically integrated our operation and expanded our manufacturing capabilities until we are now vertically integrated and buy only a few raw materials and manufacture products from those materials. As I stated above, we buy hot rolled steel coil. Even the steel mills we buy from have to use either scrap or iron ore and other products to "make" steel. We have to start with something, whether a steel mill or a grating manufacturer. I love the idea of taking a raw material and making it into something useful. We are good at that, but we have to start with raw material. On the other hand, God is not a manufacturer but a creator.

God can start with nothing and make something of it. God can also take a mess of a life and make it into something amazing. David had his heart stained with sin and shame. Psalm 51 came after David looked out of his palace and saw a woman named Bathsheba bathing. He called for her and committed adultery with her. She later informed him that she was pregnant, and since her husband was at war (fighting for David and the nation of Israel), it would be known that she was not pregnant by her husband, Uriah. To cover it up, David sent for Uriah to return from the battle and spend some time at home. Uriah came back as commanded but refused to stay in his house while his nation was fighting a battle. He would not allow himself to do that. David even went as far as getting Uriah drunk to get him to sleep with his wife, but the man still refused to sleep in his house while his fellow soldiers were in the battlefield. So David sent Uriah back to the battle with a note for Joab, his general, to attack a city, pull away from Uriah, and leave him there so he would be killed. David committed adultery and deception, attempted to cover it, and even ordered a murder. He then took Bathsheba to be his wife after her period of mourning. As if that was not bad enough, Uriah was one of David's top thirty troops who had done heroic feats for David and the children of Israel through the years. Uriah had stuck by David through the tough times.

David spent a long time trying to cover this up and was hiding from the truth. He couldn't make anything out of it. Shame was consuming his every thought.

Then the prophet Nathan came and called David out on his sin, and David repented. David knew he could cry to the Creator to make him a clean heart. "Take this sin-stained heart that my failures have tainted, and re-create that clean and pure heart I had when I was watching my father's sheep."

We can go back to Psalm 24 to recognize what qualified him to be in God's service.

> *Who shall ascend into the hill of the LORD? or who shall stand in his holy place? He that hath clean hands, and a pure heart; who hath not lifted up his soul unto vanity, nor sworn deceitfully. He shall receive the blessing from the LORD, and righteousness from the God of his salvation* (Psalm 24:3-5).

A clean hands and pure heart allowed David to ascend into the hill of the Lord and stand in His holy place. He was a recipient of God's blessing and righteousness. He now cried to God to take his sin-stained heart and make it new. He needed God to create a clean heart. He knew his heart too well and couldn't deal with it merely being washed but wanted a newly created heart put into him.

Before I move on, I have to mention 1 Corinthians 6:11, "And such were some of you: but ye are washed, but ye are sanctified, but ye are justified in the name of the Lord Jesus, and by the Spirit of our God." Paul listed all kinds of horrible things that we see in this world, sin manifested as thieves, drunkards, and other examples of our carnal nature in control of our lives. But he summed it up by saying that his audience (you and I) used to be right there. Bound by sin. Helpless to control our sinful nature. No matter how hard we tried to control our powerful fleshly nature, we couldn't do it. But we have been washed by the One who is able to create a clean heart in us. Thank God for the power of creation and His willingness to show us grace and give us a fresh start!

He is the God of the mulligan. I don't like to golf, but I do know that a mulligan is a do-over. I am so thankful He has allowed me so many mulligans in my walk with Him. I made the bad shot, the wrong decision, yet He reached into the stockpile of His grace and gave me a do-over. What an awesome God we serve! This is so important when we talk about living peaceably. It is impossible to live peaceably when we are haunted by our mistakes, but God offered Himself as one sacrifice for sin forever (Hebrews 10:12).

God gave the children of Israel a hint. He told them that He was placing two choices before them: life and death. Then comes the hint. Choose life.

> *I call heaven and earth to witness against you today, that I have set before you life and death, the blessing and the curse. So choose life in order that you may live, you and your descendants, by loving the LORD your God, by obeying His voice, and by holding fast to Him; for this is your life and the length of your days* (Deuteronomy 30:19-20, NASB).

The choice is yours. Life and death. Blessing and curse. Choose life and blessing. Do this by loving God and obeying His voice.

While we lived in Texas, Pastor Walea preached a message entitled "Making Room for Manasseh." I was writing this section of the book at the time, and it fit so well that I had to share it. Genesis 41:51, "And Joseph called the name of the firstborn Manasseh: For God, said he, hath made me forget all my toil, and all my father's house." Joseph was in Egypt and had gone through many horrible ordeals to get there. But we can sense here the deep pain that he carried with him through slavery, prison, exaltation, and abasement. Yet it wasn't prison he needed to forget. It wasn't the betrayal of Potiphar's wife or slavery. It wasn't even being forgotten by a man for whom he interpreted a dream, but it was the memory of his toil and all his father's house. Nothing can bring us more joy or pain than those we love. The pain of his father's house was still very real to Joseph. The torment, cruelty, and jealousy of his brothers haunted him in his sleep and continued to consume his thoughts. When his son was born, he was able to take the joys of becoming a parent and allow them to erase the pain of his past. I am sure he did not want to see the same issues come to his family that he experienced as a youth.

The key here is to realize that your history is no obstacle for God. Whatever God has in store for you, your history is not able to keep God from performing it in your life. You have to allow God to use you in spite of your history. He can throw our sins under the blood, but ordinarily we are the ones who struggle with God's using us because of our past. Also important is to know your current battle is no obstacle for God either. God is bigger than your past and your present. Allow God to help you forget your past and overcome your present issues so He can make you what He is desiring you to become. He is the God of fresh starts and new beginnings! You can start fresh with a healthy lifestyle today, both spiritually and naturally. Let Him do a creative work in you.

Why Christians Get Sick

"In 1976, at the age of forty-two, Dr. George Malkmus was told he had colon cancer. How could this be? He was a Christian! He was a pastor! He had dedicated his life to the Lord! His immediate response was 'Why?' But, not willing to accept this cancer as God's will for his life, he began an intensive biblical and scientific study to find out why—and to possibly find an alternative treatment to the usually unsuccessful treatments of the medical profession. What Dr. Malkmus discovered not only brought healing to his body, but also answers these questions:

"Why do Christians get sick?
"Can people be free from physical problems?
"Are cancer and other physical problems avoidable?
"What can a person do to avoid sickness?"

The above excerpt is found on the back cover of *Why Christians Get Sick* by Dr. George H. Malkmus.

Many of the questions he tackles fit well with this book. If anyone should be healthy, shouldn't it be those who have been bought with the blood of Jesus Christ and are trying to live the way He wants us to live?

Dr. Malkmus describes the amazing work of our Creator when He formed humanity from the dust of the ground—the marvelous function of the organs, the blood, our cells, and brain. He shows how different religions view sickness and the lack of knowledge among Christians in regard to health and food. In another chapter he addresses the food we eat and the problems with it. He states, "Most Christians are more concerned with the brand and grade of gasoline they put into their automobiles than they are about the quality and nutritional value of the food they put into their bodies." That is unfortunately the case for many.

He also takes a chapter to talk about the issues of legal drugs. Americans consume billions of dollars of drugs every year. These are often very unhealthy and can cause a lot of problems and health issues. He goes on to discuss the foods we eat and the stress we are under. His book deals with many of the same topics in a similar way as Stormie does in *Greater Health God's Way*.

Dr. Malkmus lists the natural laws we often ignore, but, designed by God, they can transform our lives:

1)   Pure air
2)   Pure water
3)   Pure living food (He promotes a raw vegetarian diet I don't agree with, but I believe we need to increase our intake of these foods significantly.)

4) Vigorous exercise
5) Abundant sunshine
6) Adequate rest
7) Positive thinking

I love the title of his chapter, "It's Time to Do Something about It." Our level of obedience needs to match our level of knowledge. As our understanding of healthy living grows, our behavior needs to change. Start changing habits. Study and learn what is good for you and what isn't. Set a good example. Make a difference.

Keeper of the House by Nona Freeman

Whose House?

We're given temporary residence
    In a vulnerable house of clay
    Without lease or promise of time;
    Eviction could come any day.

Since the longest residency is brief,
    How careful and wise we should be
    To occupy each short golden moment
    In the light of eternity

And nurture the clay house diligently
    Even though it came from a clod,
    For the King graces it with His presence
    To become the Temple of God.
        —Nona Freeman

Healthy Living

Nona and Bug Freeman were missionaries to Africa for forty-one years. From 1948 to 1989 they never spent a full year in the USA. When they retired, returning to America, they thought they had developed an allergy to America but realized the processing of and preservatives in the food were causing sickness. The good news is that they learned how to deal with it, and we can learn from them. At the onset of her book Nona asked:

If it is possible to:

A)   Feel better
B)   Be more productive
C)   Handle fatigue
D)   Have more stamina
E)   Minimize emotional mood swings
F)   Stimulate latent brain power and
G)   Avoid depression,

do you want to know how?
Keep reading!

In this ninety-page booklet, Nona provided some home remedies she used over the years.
Her rules for radiant health:

1)   Trust Jesus totally and give yourself to Him.
2)   Wake up every morning hungry and thirsty for God's Word, His righteousness, and His will for your life.

3) Study nutrition. Refuse to contaminate your body with food and drinks preserved with poison.

4) Drink pure water, six to eight glasses daily. Other beverages—tea, coffee, and cold drinks—do not count.

5) Exercise. Find a regimen suitable for you and stick to it.

6) Live joyfully! Commandeer your thoughts to King-worship.

7) Walk in love. Major in friendship and giving helping hands.

And the very God of peace sanctify you wholly; and I pray God your whole spirit and soul and body be preserved blameless unto the coming of our Lord Jesus Christ (1 Thessalonians 5:23).

Nona discussed the harmful foods and things we need to avoid, to take care of our clay house! I recommend this booklet, an easy read to keep awareness of our health in our conscious minds.

As a side note. . . .

I have heard of a number of people whom God was drawing to commit their lives to Him and get into church, yet they did not want to because they have seen too many people get into church, gain weight, and fail to take care of themselves. They did not want to do that or have that happen to them. There are many struggles for the new convert when he or she wants to get into church, but that shouldn't be one of them. The church needs to rise up in the area of health. It would help us reach a world that is lost but health-conscious. We would be more effective as well. Healthy living gives you more energy and a sharper mind. It is worth the effort. We are of far more value to the kingdom of God when we are healthy than when we are sick.

The Balance and Aging

I want to age gracefully. We can't stop aging, but we can eliminate thorns in our life that cause premature aging. It is not too late to start getting healthier. We see "Biggest Loser" type testimonials about people losing a bunch of weight and getting their lives back. It is far better to avoid gaining all that weight in the first place. But even if you are already really out of shape, just start small and work on it every day.

John Maxwell has something he calls the principle of five. If you need to cut down a huge tree, take an ax, hit the tree five times, and do that every day. Abraham Lincoln said if he had four hours to chop down a tree, he would spend the first three hours sharpening his ax. Based on those two thoughts, I propose that preparation and consistency are the real keys. You can reach your goal, but you need to do a little bit every day and prepare for what you are about to face.

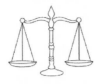

Chapter Five

Thorns

As the apostle Paul wrote to the church at Corinth, he opened himself to criticism and speculation by penning the following words:

> *And lest I should be exalted above measure through the abundance of the revelations, there was given to me a thorn in the flesh, the messenger of Satan to buffet me, lest I should be exalted above measure. For this thing I besought the Lord thrice, that it might depart from me. And he said to me, My grace is sufficient for thee: for my strength is made perfect in weakness. Most gladly therefore will I rather glory in my infirmities, that the power of Christ may rest upon me. Therefore I take pleasure in infirmities, in reproaches, in necessities, in persecutions, in distresses for*

Christ's sake: for when I am weak, then am I strong (2 Corinthians 12:7-10).

Consider all the epistles he wrote, all of those to whom he ministered, those who were healed by the apostle's hand, those who were inspired and touched, those he had prayed through to the Holy Ghost, and the miracles that were wrought by his prayers and hands. We recall all of those things, yet the Lord gave him a thorn lest he should be exalted above measure.

The below excerpt is from an article by J. Mark Jordan in the *Ohio Apostolic News*.

> It sneaks through the back door of your consciousness; it looms before your tightly closed eyes in prayer; it pulls you down each time you take a step up; it laughs at your attempts at discipleship; it hollows out your achievements, voids your victories and ridicules your goals. No amount of fasting, prayer, study, counseling, rebuke, or encouragement matters. It's always there. It is your thorn.

A thorn is defined as a stiff, sharp-pointed, straight or curved woody projection on the stem or other part of a plant. It is the part of a rose that keeps us from grabbing it. On plants it works as a protective agent for the plant. It can be a stake for impaling, a surgical instrument, the point of a fishhook, something that causes severe pain or constant irritation.

I have fallen in the woods and had a thorn go deep in my hand. I have had a thorn stick in my pants leg and irritate me as I walked until I could remove it. I have had thorns scratch and tear my arms and legs while clearing land or working in the woods. Thorns don't always cause severe pain or cause major issues, but they are a constant irritant that drives you crazy until you can remove them. Paul stated, "There was given to me a thorn in the flesh . . . to buffet me." That doesn't sound like fun.

Centuries of speculation have discussed Paul's thorn. Was it cataracts, epileptic seizures, earaches, headaches, malaria, rheumatism, reoccurring nightmares, depression, a divorce, or relationship problems? You can search the commentaries, listen to and read messages from history, and hear a lot of theories on what the thorn could be. I even heard someone say it could have been bed-wetting! In Galatians 4:15 (NASB) Paul said, "For I bear you witness, that, if possible, ye would have plucked out your eyes and given them to me." Some think this is an indication that Paul may have been blind.

Honestly, who knows what the thorn that Paul talked about was? Or maybe we should ask who cares what the thorn was? Does it matter what the thorn was? I am sure that Paul cared!

"There was given to me a thorn." It caused severe pain at a maximum or constant irritation at a minimum, as well as twenty centuries of speculation. We do not know what it was, but we do know one of the greatest Christians of all times had one. It is interesting that Paul could have told us what it was that was irritating him and causing him pain, but he chose not to tell us. One thing is certain, though. Something troubled Paul, and God did not take it away.

Usually people say a lot by not saying anything! Did he not tell to save his ministry, to save embarrassment, to keep from throwing meat to the dogs? The religious Jews would have had something at which to throw jabs. Something troubled Paul continually, and God did not take it away. Paul prayed three times for deliverance, but God gently but firmly said no. What if it was a mental illness? An apostle dealing with depression would be a problem. Would he have been canonized if he had persistent nightmares? What if Paul struggled with something unspeakable or taboo for an apostle to deal with? He saw many healed at his own hand and by his prayers. Yet he couldn't get the answer he wanted from God for this issue.

Thorns! "Deliver me" was his cry to God, but the reply was a firm but compassionate no. As his pain increased, so did the available grace. That is always the case. As pain goes up, so does grace. If we look to God, He will meet us at the point of our need. Great spiritual exploits, missionary journeys galore, and the authorship of the majority of the New Testament, all came with a troubling thorn. Yet that thorn made him who he was. Paul prayed three times to be delivered, and all three times God said no.

I view Paul's three noted prayers for deliverance to be more than just mentioning the thorn in his prayer before a gathering of the saints, but I envision his three specific prayers for deliverance to be more like times when he locked himself in and spent some focused time praying for deliverance and healing once and for all. Focused, intense prayer and fasting went out about the thorn. Three times he locked himself in with one purpose in mind. "Deliver me from my thorn." He wrestled with God as Jacob wrestled with the angel by Jabbok in Genesis 32, not letting go until he got an answer. Each time the answer came back as no.

When God says no, what a challenging time it is to continue to trust God when He gives you no for the answer, the opposite of what you want to hear. Therefore, Paul had to factor the thorn into his life. If God doesn't take it away, I will have to learn how to deal with it. "I will have to learn how to trust You when You don't answer my prayer and I have to continue to deal with the thorn." But as pain increased, so did the grace!

I seldom know why God doesn't always answer the way we want Him to, but I do know that "now we see through a glass darkly," but someday we will see clearly what God was doing in our lives. The thorn tempered Paul's divine revelations, prevented pride from destroying him, and keenly honed his dependence on God. It perfected him with God's strength rather than allowing him to depend on his own. By refusing to identify his thorn, he focused our attention on what it did rather than what it was.

God designed thorns to be catalysts for perfection. If we fail to see the value of our thorn, we will never achieve the anointing that the thorn can bring. God does not always remove the thorn from our lives because He knows that sometimes we need the thorn. Sometimes the thorn makes us what He wants us to be. But He doesn't abandon you when He has a thorn in you; He just gives you the grace you need to get through that moment. How many times have people dealt with stuff, and at that moment God's grace kicked in? We may think we cannot handle a miscarriage, the death of a family member, or a bout with cancer, but a year later we can look back and see how God carried us through those times in our lives. Pain increased, and so did grace. In the balance between pain and grace, the balance always tips in our favor in the hand of God. He knows exactly the extent of our limits in dealing with a thorn, and He does not put too much on that balance, no more than we can handle. When affliction increases in our life, He puts more grace on the other side to balance it.

This man Paul, who wrought great works for God, did all those things with a throbbing thorn. It kept him depending on God's strength, not on his own. Paul kept his attention on what it did and not on what it was. Even though your thorn will probably be different from his thorn, know its purpose and how to handle it because we will all have to deal with thorns. We see natural imperfections and challenges, but God designed thorns to bring perfection to us. In our failure to see the value of a thorn, we will never achieve the level of anointing we could have achieved by dealing with the thorn and growing because of it. We have to see the value of a thorn.

In *Wreck My Life*, Mo Isom states, "What if hearing and accepting the hardest things is exactly what sets us free? What if we began to recognize trouble and adversity as sacred rather than scarring? As promised rather than game-changing? As purposeful rather than punishing? What if we truly believed there was purpose in our pain and a plan in our persecution? What would our world look like if we shifted our mentality and began to rejoice in our adversity, knowing adversity produces perseverance, perseverance produces character, and character produces hope? (See Romans 5:3-5.)"

She goes on to say, "In a broken world, our adversity and suffering will not cease but our perspective can boldly shift. We can begin to embrace adversity in a new light. We can begin to surrender the pain and suffering of our past, accept the forgiveness and grace offered in the present, and invite a holy God to wreck our lives. To unhinge the lies we've believed, to shake our preconceived ideas and beliefs, to obliterate our bondage and our shame and our pride and our defeat. With radical, unshakable faith placed in a radical, unfailing King, we are able to appreciate the wreckage of our past and orchestrate the voluntary wreckage of our future for the glory of a King who was first wrecked on our behalf."

Jesus said:

You're blessed when you're at the end of your rope. With less of you there is more of God and his rule. You're blessed when you feel you've lost what is most dear to you. Only then can you be embraced by the One most dear to you. . . . You're blessed when your commitment to God provokes persecution. The persecution drives you even deeper into God's kingdom. Not only that—count yourselves blessed every time people put you down or throw you out or speak lies about you to discredit me. What it means is that the truth is too close for comfort and they are uncomfortable. You can be glad when that happens—give a cheer, even!—for though they don't like it, I do! And all heaven applauds. And know that you are in good company. My prophets and witnesses have always gotten into this kind of trouble (Matthew 5:3-4, 10-12, *The Message*).

Tough conditions make tough people. Paul wrote in Galatians 6:17 (RSV), "Henceforth let no man trouble me; for I bear on my body the marks of Jesus." Thorns shape our lives into the image of Christ.

Strength requires stress for development. Power comes from resistance. "For two years, scientists sequestered themselves in an artificial environment called Biosphere Two. Inside their self-sustaining community, the Biospherians created a number of mini-environments, including a desert, rainforest, even an ocean. Nearly every weather condition could be simulated except one, wind. Over time, the effects of their windless environment became apparent. A number of acacia trees bent over and even snapped. Without the stress of wind to strengthen the wood, the trunks grew weak and could not hold up their own weight" (Jay Akkerman, *Leadership*). Tough conditions make tough people.

Philip Harrelson says, "Could it be that the thorn was what shaped his life into the image of Christ? No man will arrive in heaven without some scars that life places upon him. But the scars of life should mark us in the manner of a Cross. The thorns shape our lives into the image of Christ."

In Daniel 5 we find one of the most bizarre stories in the Scripture. The royal household was having a party when abruptly a hand showed up and wrote on the wall. That would completely freak me out. In the *God's Word* version it says that King Belshazzar "turned pale, and his thoughts frightened him. His hip joints became loose, and his knees knocked against each other." After going through the process of calling Daniel in so he could tell them the meaning, the king got a message: "TEKEL: You have been weighed in the balances, and found wanting" (Daniel 5:27, NKJV). You have been weighed in the balances. His marks are on one side, and your attitude is on the other. Unfortunately, you have been found deficient, lacking, and wanting. The *God's Word* version says, "You have been put on a scale and found to be too light." "King," God said, "I put you in the balance, and when I put you in the balance, it bottomed out and not in your favor."

Thorns have roses. What did God say to Job? In my words, He said, "I have put him in the balances, and he has tipped the scales in My favor." God's balances are accurate. When Job found himself in the balances, they sunk on the side of God and elevated on the side of his fleshly desires. What was the devil's response? "You haven't given him any thorns." Let some thorns come with his rosebush, and let's see what kind of balance he finds himself in.

Then we read the next thirty-five chapters of the balance his friends tried to put him in while Job defended himself against their accusations. "Who is righteous?" he would say. "Where is God?" He found himself consistently trying to figure out the balances of God. But we will never understand the balances of God because my righteousness will get me nowhere when I find myself in God's scale. But what Job finally concluded was that it wasn't about his righteousness at all but about what God was trying to do in him.

Job said, "Is there not a mediator?" When the balance starts to tip because of thorns, God's grace comes to push on the other side to bring you back into balance. That is the beauty of the balances of God. Proverbs says that God doesn't like a rigged balance when you are trading. Don't use rigged balances. But God always uses a rigged balance in our favor because of the element of grace. We find in these balances His marks on one side and our attitude on the other. What will you do with the thorn—be bitter or be marked with His image? Your attitude determines what you will do with any thorns that God has placed or allowed in your life.

Some people get so stuck on the thorn God places in them that they never do anything more than get bitter about the thorn instead of allowing it to conform them into the image of Christ. The process of dealing with the thorn is what really has the power to transform us. How will you handle your thorn? Will you be found wanting, or will you tip the scales on the side of God's favor?

How do you know when to pray and fast and keep praying and fasting? Paul stopped at three times. The

Scripture teaches us to keep asking, seeking, and knocking. The woman who was dealing with the unrighteous judge and the man who asked his neighbor for bread were commended for their perseverance, but Paul said, "Most gladly I will rather boast in my infirmities, that the power of Christ may rest upon me. Therefore I take pleasure in infirmities, in reproaches, in needs, in persecutions, in distresses, for Christ's sake. For when I am weak, then I am strong" (NKJV).

Which is it? Keep praying for the answer you want, or stop praying and boast in your infirmities? It can be extremely frustrating when praying for God to use you and then getting stuck in the frustration of a holding pattern. How does this all fit? The Word of God is without contradiction, so there has to be an answer for this.

A paradox is a seemingly self-contradictory statement that is actually true. The Bible has a number of perplexing paradoxes. James said, "Humble yourselves in the sight of the Lord, and he shall lift you up." How does that make sense? The Lord despises a proud look. "God resisteth the proud, but giveth grace unto the humble." Isaiah spoke of Lucifer's exalting himself and being cast out of heaven, yet Christ humbled Himself and took on the form of a man. It was a paradox of exaltation through humility, and destruction through pride.

Another paradox is receiving through giving. Give, and ye shall receive. I remember hearing worship leaders pray for an offering, asking God to bless those who have to give and those who have not. This is not a biblical prayer. God blesses the giver. You have something to give because you give. It is a true test of your faith to give, and God has proven over and over that He blesses those who give. Give abundantly of your time, talent, and material possessions, and God will bless you abundantly. Other biblical paradoxes include freedom through servitude, gain by loss, finding through losing, and living through dying.

The last paradox I want to touch on is strength through weakness. Paul stated, "I take pleasure in infirmities, in reproaches, in necessities, in persecutions, in distresses for Christ's sake: for when I am weak, then I am strong" (NKJV). We want the world to see the power of Christ in us, but His power is displayed in the midst of our weakness. The struggles and trials provide the times when God can show Himself strong in us. The Word of God is not in conflict, but these seeming contradictions reveal powerful truths found in God's Word and how they display His influence and power in our lives.[1]

I have heard that we need to be as tough as nails and as pliable as gold. Sometimes God does not heal when we ask Him to heal. When I was pastoring we had a guest speaker preach about an outrageous God and healing one week, and the next week we needed to guard our attitudes when He did not heal a young mother who died of cancer. Our attitude makes the difference. As life dishes out its challenges, we often bounce between frustrations and defeat and joy and victory.

> *Have this attitude in yourselves which was also in Christ Jesus: who, although He existed in the form of God, did not regard equality with God a thing to be grasped,*

but emptied himself, taking the form of a bond-servant, and being made in the likeness of men. Being found in appearance as a man, He humbled Himself by becoming obedient to the point of death, even death on a cross (Philippians 2:5-8, NASB).

We are to allow the same humility, brokenness, and sacrifice Jesus showed to evidence itself in us. It is easy to trust God when everything is going right, but when everything seems to be going against us, we truly see how much we trust Him.

Job uttered these words in the midst of his trial:

Look, I go forward, but He is not there,
And backward, but I cannot perceive Him;
When He works on the left hand, I cannot behold Him,
When He turns to the right hand, I cannot see Him.
But He knows the way that I take;
When He has tested me, I shall come forth as gold.
My foot has held fast to His steps;
I have kept His way and not turned aside.
I have not departed from the commandment of His lips;
I have treasured the words of His mouth
More than my necessary food
(Job 23:8-12, NKJV, my emphasis).

"Have you considered my servant Job?" I believe I would rather not have God consider me. The process of refinement is the potter's wheel or a desert detour. He will push and prod and poke and then put you in the fire, and when He gets done, He says, "Now I can do something with him." It is like gold that is tried in fire again and again until the final product is pure and ready for use. Trusting God to make of you what He wants of you is what puts you on the potter's wheel. Usually during these times it seems God is nowhere to be found. Job and David both wrote of their search for God in the front and back and to the right and to the left, yet they could not find any help. But in the midst of one of the hardest trials anyone has ever faced, as if God had abandoned him, Job acknowledged, "When I get through this test, I am going to come forth as gold." Purified, pliable, and usable in the hands of God.

Another pathway to promise is when God sends you on a desert detour.

> *Where is the* LORD *that brought us up out of the land of Egypt,* that led us *through the* wilderness, *through a land of* deserts *and of* pits, *through a* land of drought, *and of the* shadow of death, *through a land that no man passed through, and where no man dwelt? And I brought you into a plentiful country, to eat the fruit thereof and the goodness thereof; but when ye entered, ye defiled my land, and made mine heritage an abomination* (Jeremiah 2:6-7, my emphases).

The path to the promise is often rough and desolate. We often couldn't handle the promise if we did not have to take the road that took us where the promise is. Desert detours are the routes God takes us from promise to fulfillment. Let's look at a few examples of desert detours in the Scripture.

Joseph had God-given dreams about the day his brothers would bow before him. Before he could get to that place and see this promise fulfilled, his brothers threw him in a pit, stole his coat, and then sold him into slavery. He ended up in jail and later as a leader in a foreign land. He had to take a massive desert detour. One mind-boggling fact about Joseph's desert detour is that he was thrown into prison because of his integrity. He was sold into slavery for telling the dreams that were given to him by God, and we don't see an occasion when Joseph had any lapse in integrity. We usually like to tie a desert place to someone's lapse of integrity. But we see time and again in the Scripture that people go on a desert detour for no fault of their own.

Somewhere in the desert Joseph forgot his dream. Then God brought it back to him. God had given him a promise, and Joseph had to get to the place where God needed him to be to fulfill the promise that God had for him. Yet in the midst of a multi-year detour, he did not lose his integrity. God used the detour to get him in the right place. God's plan for Joseph included an extensive desert detour, but at the end of the detour the promise was fulfilled.

Moses spent forty years in Pharaoh's house and then forty years on the back side of a desert. Then he had to lead the children of Israel through the desert for another forty years. He had to take more than one desert detour, but he started off with a temper so severe that he murdered someone in a fit of rage. After his desert detour he became known as the meekest man on earth. He actually talked God into showing mercy. That he could reach the point of talking God into showing mercy has always amazed me. This is the same guy who had an anger issue before his desert detour. I would consider that extreme mercy. After fleeing from Egypt, Moses spent forty years on the back side of the desert. God used those forty years to make the man, to develop the attributes and characteristics in Moses so that he would be able to lead the children of Israel out of Egypt and to the Promised Land.

Moses had a detour to lead the children of Israel as part of his desert trek, but that was also their desert detour. They marched out of Egypt as free people for the first time in hundreds of years and then spent forty years wandering in the wilderness. Moses would have wiped out the entire nation when God gave him the option if he had not spent forty years prior tending sheep. If anyone deserved the Promised Land, it had to be Moses. Yet he was denied because he had a flashback to the old man when he smote the rock in anger. This detour for the entire nation was important to get the attitude of Egypt out of the children of Israel. It was not enough for them to get out of the location or even to be delivered from slavery. God had to get Egypt out of them and not just get them out of Egypt.

Joseph's detour was to get him on location and in position to save the children of Israel when famine hit, but Moses' detour helped him to have the right characteristics to lead the children of Israel out of bondage and not kill them all. God used a detour to get Egypt out of the children of Israel and get them into the Promised Land.

Joseph—to get the right person in the right position
Moses—to get the right character in the right person
Israel—to get the wrong attitude out of the right people

Where does He have you?

John the Baptist started with a promise from way back in the Book of Isaiah, "The voice of him that crieth in the wilderness."

> *In those days John the Baptist came preaching in the wilderness of Judea, and saying, "Repent, for the kingdom of heaven is at hand!" For this is he who was spoken of by the prophet Isaiah, saying: "The voice of one crying in the wilderness: 'Prepare the way of the LORD; Make His paths straight.' " Now John himself was clothed in camel's hair, with a leather belt around his waist; and his food was locusts and wild honey. Then Jerusalem, all Judea, and all the region around the Jordan went out to him and were baptized by him in the Jordan, confessing their sins* (Matthew 3:1-6, NKJV).

> *And the child grew, and waxed strong in spirit, and was in the deserts till the day of his shewing unto Israel* (Luke 1:80).

John the Baptist had a detour ministry. Rough, crude, rugged, and direct were all words to describe the ministry of John the Baptist. He was six months older than Jesus, growing up in the deserts until "the day of his shewing."

He was the one paving the way for Jesus. He conducted the first baptismal services in the muddy Jordan River. He came preaching a doctrine never heard before, that of repentance and baptism, setting the stage for the One whose shoes he wasn't worthy to unloose. Yet he would baptize Jesus.

He delivered a bold and direct message. He grew up in the wilderness and preached from there. That is some kind of power! He did not go to the people, but the people came to him.

After about six months of ministry, he baptized Jesus and shortly thereafter was thrown in prison. After some time (some believe almost three years), his head was chopped off. The disciples buried his headless body.

This was probably not the path to promise he expected: scorned, jailed, and beheaded. But that is where God had him. He was born in the hillside and grew up in the desert to prepare him for the job he was to do.

His entire ministry was a detour ministry. He was the forerunner, the one who laid the ax to the root of the tree and stirred things up in preparation for Jesus' coming. This is why we read in Matthew 11:12 (ISV), "From the days of John the Baptist until the present, the kingdom of heaven has been forcefully advancing, and violent people have been attacking it." He lived in the desert wilderness and was a total outcast. A desert detour prepared the way for the Savior.

Jesus, before He fired up the miracle machine, spent forty days in the wilderness in prayer and fasting. Jesus was the original child of promise. He was born with promise. He was promise fulfilled, the Word that became flesh, the plan that was embodied. He was our perfect example, yet we see the Spirit driving Him into the wilderness for a forty-day detour. Was the purpose of this detour, like with Joseph, to get the right person at the right place at the right time? No. Was it comparable to Moses, to get the right qualities in the right person? No. Was it like the nation of Israel to get the right attitude in the right people? No. Jesus was on location, was the promise, had the right attitude, and was the right person. He was at the point, though, where it was necessary for Him to prepare Himself. These times of preparation are examples for us.

> *It came to pass in those days that Jesus came from Nazareth of Galilee, and was baptized by John in the Jordan. And immediately, coming up from the water, He saw the heavens parting and the Spirit descending upon Him like a dove. Then a voice came from heaven, "You are My beloved Son, in whom I am well pleased."* Immediately the Spirit drove Him into the wilderness. *And He was there in the wilderness* forty days, *tempted by Satan, and was with the wild beasts; and the angels ministered to* Him (Mark 1:9-13, NKJV, my emphases).

Those willing to follow the Spirit into the desert detours are great examples for us. How many desert detours that last years could we avoid if we took some intentional desert detours? Immediately after the forty days in the wilderness to pray and fast, Jesus was confronted with temptation directly from the devil. He might not have been able to stand during the temptation if He had not tapped into the source of power while on the detour through the wilderness.

He also endured the deaths of John the Baptist, Lazarus, and probably Joseph, His earthly father figure. He got his strength to go through these tough times by taking a voluntary desert detour.

The battle at Calvary was won in the Garden of Gethsemane. Probably the trip in the wilderness helped Him get through some of the other trials in His life.

What does the path to promise look like? The path, the timing, and the route look more like you expect because they are voluntary. This involves willingly saying, "God, I am going to set things aside so I can get in touch with You and tap into the source of my strength."

Then God said to Jacob, "Arise, go up to Bethel and dwell there; and make an altar there to God, who appeared to you when you fled from the face of Esau your brother." And Jacob said to his household and to all who were with him, "Put away the foreign gods that are among you, purify yourselves, and change your garments. Then let us arise and go up to Bethel; and

I will make an altar there to God, who answered me in the day of my distress and has been with me in the way which I have gone" (Genesis 35:1-3, NKJV).

We see God calling Jacob to get his household in order. Get ready for a time of preparation and calling. You can read further in this account that God also put terror in the people of the land for Jacob. God will provide wherever He guides. Voluntary desert detours are usually much shorter in duration, yet you come out with the strength you need. A time of prayer, fasting, the Word, and worship brings down spiritual strongholds and prepares you for the promise God has in store for you.

John's desert detour was early in his ministry. John was accustomed to the desert because he placed himself there, and when he needed to fulfill his role as the voice of one crying in the wilderness, he was able to do so because he had already accepted that detour. Our voluntary detour examples show that the route was the right route because they set themselves apart for a season in His service. Get away, focus on Him, and see if He doesn't open doors for you.

Are these detours just for people in the Bible days, or do we sometimes have to take detours on our path to the promise? The challenge is staying on the path in the midst of these detours and not getting too frustrated in the process. Never quit, and never give up.

Let us take a look at Mary and Joseph. "Okay," God said, "you are the ones I will use when I robe Myself in flesh and come to this earth, but with all of these prophecies I moved on the prophets to deliver, how will I get you in the right place at the right time? You meet the qualifications, but I need you to be in Bethlehem at the right time to fulfill My promise." Roman rule, the right bloodline, the right characteristics and habits, and then the census, all fell into place in His perfect timing. If the promise said the Prince of Peace, the everlasting Father, and the mighty God was to be born, why am I looking in a manger for that promise to be fulfilled? It was painful, it was not easy, they were poor, they were dirty, and the world was a mess.

What about Joseph, the son of Jacob (Israel)? The dream foretold that his family would bow to him, but they hated him. "In a certain year there will be famine, and I will need someone on location at the right time to deliver My people. I told Abraham that his seed would be in Egypt for four hundred years. How am I going to get them delivered from the famine and in Egypt, from the land of promise to bondage and then back to the land of promise?" God used Joseph's desert detour to set things up for the fulfillment of the prophecy.

It may not look like you anticipated it to look. This doesn't look like what I thought the promise would look like. Joseph's dream said they were supposed to bow to him. "I didn't figure it meant while they were throwing me in a pit. Pastures, pits, Potiphar, and prisons weren't what the promise was supposed to look like." But that is what it looked like.

The timing—It just "so happened" that those Ishmaelite traders came through that exact pasture at that time, and they were headed to Egypt. Isn't it somewhat ironic that God used Ishmaelite traders to handle the delivery? The Ishmael mess was Abraham's way of helping God fulfill His impossible promise. "Since God can't do it, I will have to get it done." But the promise isn't for our manipulation; it is for God to do. The difference between God's timing and ours is usually drastic.

The route—Joseph didn't like the route that God took. That desert detour was long, painful, and embarrassing and separated him from his family, but it was the will of God. The path that Abraham took was also grueling. With the promise of a child, he and Sarah just kept getting older. Then he was told to sacrifice that child on a mountain. God asked him to surrender the very promise he had been given. Sometimes the route is the test that we need for God to use us and make us what He wants us to be. A desert detour.

That desert detour may be your salvation. It may be the salvation of someone else. Don't get frustrated with God's timing, the look, or the route He takes you on the road to promise.

In *Wreck My Life*, Mo Isom recalls the feeling she should try out for the LSU football team as a kicker. She spent eighteen months working out and dealing with the scrutiny of the media. She had been a star soccer player and was a tremendous athlete. She was able to kick fifty-three-yard field goals and felt she was lined up to make the team. Then she was cut. She was told no to that portion of her dream. She had been a student athlete for the past four years so it was more than just being cut. It was a change in her identity. After the 'no' she said, "I was called to listen to God's leading, take on the challenge

He presented me, and passionately pursue the goal He set, in Christ's name. I was never assured of the result. Would I have been as willing to take on such a crazy, vulnerable, and challenging feat had I known there was a closed door at the end? No. Yet God had reasons for every step of my journey." She went on to say, "Was I a failure for having received a no? No. *The success was not in the outcome but in the steps of faith it took to complete the journey.*" Her desert detour helped to mold and guide her on her journey and prepare her for the next steps God had in store for her.

> *The wilderness and the wasteland shall be glad for them, And* the desert shall rejoice *and* blossom *as the rose; It shall blossom abundantly and rejoice, Even with joy and singing.* . . . Strengthen *the weak hands, And* make firm *the feeble knees. Say to those who are* fearful-hearted, *"Be strong, do not fear! Behold, your God will come with vengeance, With the recompense of God; He will come and save you."* Then *the eyes of the blind shall be opened, And the ears of the deaf shall be unstopped. Then the lame shall leap like a deer, And the tongue of the dumb sing. For* waters shall burst forth in the wilderness, *And* streams in the desert. The parched ground shall become a pool, *And the thirsty land springs of water; In the habitation of jackals, where each lay, There shall be*

grass with reeds and rushes. A highway shall be there, and a road, And it shall be called the Highway of Holiness. *The unclean shall not pass over it, But it shall be for others.* Whoever walks the road, although a fool, Shall not go astray. *No lion shall be there, Nor shall any ravenous beast go up on it; It shall not be found there.* But the redeemed shall walk there, And the ransomed of the LORD shall return, *And come to Zion with singing, With everlasting joy on their heads.* They shall obtain joy and gladness, *And sorrow and sighing shall flee away* (Isaiah 35:1-10, NKJV, my emphases).

We are parched ground but have been redeemed and ransomed. God calls us to encourage and strengthen ourselves and others, and the end result should be our praise and rejoicing. There is no lion there. Your adversary the devil is like a roaring lion going about, seeking whom he may devour, but he can't touch you any longer. You need to declare to him, "Can't touch this. I'm on the Highway of Holiness; I have been redeemed." You see, it is not about what we have done, because we are saved by grace; we have been redeemed. We have been placed on the highway of holiness, on a journey in pursuit of Him and ever drawing closer to Him—be ye holy for I am holy—in our walk and life and thought.

God's desire is not for us to die in the wilderness or to leave the caravan in the middle of the desert but to stay on the path so He can bring the promise that He desires to give us. He is not slack concerning His promise, but these detours we need make it hard. Give us the strength, Lord, to stay on course when we get stuck in a detour. The fine balance between accepting the thorn and praying for deliverance is recognizing what God is trying to do in you in the process.

"Let this mind be in you, which was also in Christ Jesus" (Philippians 2:5). We must maintain an attitude of humility and submission even while in the desert.

Nothing we can face compares to the cross He had to face. There is no thorn we could have that compares with His crown of thorns. Even if you faced a literal cross that was the same that Jesus endured, it would not equal what He went through because of two things:

1. While you would be powerless to stop the process, He wasn't. That is a big difference. He could have removed any of the thorns that He had to deal with, but He did not so that we could be victorious.
2. He was sinless but bore on the cross the weight of all sins past, present, and future.

He took on those things, and we take on His image. When we take on His image, we take on some pain and suffering so we can come from trials as faithful. The balance, it is all about relationship and worship. Our attitude stops us from even tampering with the things that would show us to be unfaithful. Everyone knows stories about the spoiled brat who was handed everything and does not know how to handle anything because he never had to handle any thorns. Thorns are critical for our full spiritual development. I hate to say it, but the will of God sometimes brings adversity. Adversity that knocks on your door is a tremendous test of your attitude, but if you keep your attitude right and keep your focus on Him, when you come out on the other side you will come out tried and as precious as gold. He can't use you until you go through the process.

Self-inflicted Thorns

The Bible also tells us about self-inflicted thorns. My parents always had a garden when I was a child. My dad would till the garden, and then my mom would plant the garden. We never planted weeds in the garden, but they always appeared. My sister and I had to help weed the garden. I hated weeding the garden, the flowerbeds, or anything else. I have done my best to avoid that task as much as possible as an adult. Thankfully, my wife enjoys working in the flowerbeds, and as long as I help with the heavier manual labor, she takes care of the beautiful flowerbeds at our house. Weeds just seem to appear, just like thorns show up in our lives. But at times we put the thorns in our lives.

> *The angel of the LORD went up from Gilgal to Bokim and said to the Israelites, "I brought you out of Egypt into this land that I swore to give your ancestors, and I said I would never break my covenant with*

you. For your part, you were not to make any covenants with the people living in this land; instead, you were to destroy their altars. But you disobeyed my command. Why did you do this? So now I declare that I will no longer drive out the people living in your land. They will be thorns in your sides, and their gods will be a constant temptation to you." When the angel of the LORD finished speaking, the people wept loudly. So they called the place Bokim (which means "weeping"), and they offered sacrifices there to the LORD (Judges 2:1-5, NLT).

For a graduation present for my son, we went on an aoudad hunt. An aoudad is a mountain goat originally from Africa that was introduced to the desert mountainous areas of Texas. This is in the western side of Texas on the Mexican border. It is some of the roughest land I have ever experienced. Everything there is an extreme, overwhelmingly dry, with little annual rainfall. When it does rain, it pours and causes flash floods. It was not uncommon to wake up with the temperature in the low 40s and then a few hours later realize it was in the 90s. Everything that grows in this harsh region has something that will poke, stab, or poison you. We chose to go on that hunt. Harsh conditions, free-range animals, and a challenging week, all the aspects of that time with my son thrilled me. We created memories that will last a lifetime, and my son got a nice ram that will be mounted in his home someday and will be a talking point for years to come.

During that hunt I stepped on thorns that went all the way through the two-inch soles of my hunting boots. We all had cuts on our legs and arms. Some wounds were from poisonous plants, and the affected area would swell up and hurt. We compared wounds each night and talked about the pain and how tough it was, but the bottom line is we chose to put those thorns in our path.

That is precisely what the children of Israel did as well. God promised them that He would be in covenant with them and would give them the land. He would be their God, and they would be His people. But God's promises are usually conditional promises. If/then promises are the norm with God. If my people . . . then I will . . . is how God usually operates. The promises are awesome, but the commitment runs parallel with the promise. God told them not to make any covenants with the people of the land. They should destroy the altars of these pagan gods and not intermarry with the unbelievers. They did not do their part and decided instead to walk into the thorn patch in front of them. Unfortunately, the people they refused to destroy were to become the thorns in their sides, thorns they chose to dwell with.

The people wept. How many times do we make choices that end up becoming thorns in our sides and then weep over the result of our own decisions? We choose what to eat, whether to sleep or exercise, whether to pray or play, whether to read the Word or something that will fuel desires we should avoid, and then we weep over the consequences of our decisions. We may place voluntary thorns in our lives, yet many times these thorns destroy us. So much depends on the choices we make.

Now that I have been a parent for many years, I realize how little I know about the subject of parenting. I try to be consistent and understanding while drawing firm lines with consequences when crossed. I recently saw this quote on a sign at a gas station (Bucee's for those of you from Texas): "While we try to teach our children all about life, our children teach us what life is all about."

One day when I was particularly frustrated with one of our children, it hit me just how much that one was acting like me. It is haunting to feel such anger and hear the tender voice of God saying, "Where do you think he got that from?" Then it hits me like a ton of bricks that he is doing exactly what I would have done. F. J. Ellis would always say, "What you do in moderation, your children will do in excess." The thorns we place in our lives may not destroy us, but they may end up destroying our children. Guard yourself from thorns that you can avoid. Never ignore the voice of God or godly counsel in your life.

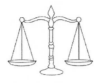

Chapter Six

Mental Illness

T his section is very challenging. Also, the subject is rarely touched in the church world. Few in the church are willing to address mental illness. We have been fans of *Focus on the Family*'s "Adventures in Odyssey" for many years. The radio program centers on a wise, older Christian man named John Avery Whitaker, who goes by the name Whit. He owns and operates an ice cream and discovery emporium called Whit's End. The program has been around since the late '80s, and the characters are consistent. Our family has grown up with the characters. The program is full of wonderful spiritual insights and life lessons.

One of the main characters is an old farmer named Tom Riley. Tom and his wife had a son, Timmy, but Tom's wife died of cancer. Tom remarried a lady named Agnes. Timmy died in a boating accident, and Agnes was unable to bear children. Soon after Timmy died, Agnes was admitted to a mental hospital due to the depression that overwhelmed her. For years Tom's wife was not mentioned, and the program rarely indicates that Tom is even married. Then album 28, in an episode entitled "The Other Woman," introduces the listener to his wife.

Tom is the mayor of Odyssey, and Bart Rathbone wants to discourage him from running for re-election so he has a better chance to be elected. Bart and his family get pictures of Tom Riley sitting on a bench with a unknown woman at the Hillendale Haven Mental Health Center. The local papers print the picture as if it is a huge scandal. Reality is that the mysterious woman is his wife, and the so-called scandal was actually Tom sitting with his wife. He ends up deciding not to run for mayor and holds a press conference to let the community know that the pictures are of his wife, she suffers from a mental illness, and she has been hospitalized for many years.

Tom tells his friends that his "wife suffers from a mental illness, a deep depression that keeps her from being able to cope with all the pressures that others take for granted." Toward the end of the program, some of his friends who didn't know anything about his wife discussed why he had never asked them to pray for his wife. Whit mentions that when she first went to the hospital, Tom would mention it in church and request prayer, "but no one knew what to do or how to respond. At first they prayed for her healing, but she just didn't get any better. It was awkward and eventually people stopped asking Tom about it and Tom stopped mentioning it." The discussion continues and Whit tells Eugene (one of his employees), "A lot of Christians have a hard time dealing with unanswered prayer, and problems like mental illness make it even messier for us." Whit says that the various forms of mental illness are very complex and not easily fixed. At times God heals it immediately, sometimes He takes His time, and sometimes He doesn't heal at all. His reasons are His own. This enigma leaves us stuck with the frailty of our humanness, dependent on the power of God's will, and obliged to keep praying hard. They go on to discuss Horatio Spafford.

Horatio Spafford was the author of the powerful song, "It Is Well with my Soul." Two years after scarlet fever took their young son from them in 1873, the Spaffords decided to spend the holiday in England with his friend, D. L. Moody. Due to a business delay, Horatio's wife and four children sailed ahead of him. On November 22, 1873, an iron sailing vessel struck the steamship *Ville du Havre*, and 226 people, including their four daughters, perished at sea.

His wife sent Spafford a telegram, "Saved alone." Spafford immediately sailed to England, and while over the location of his daughters' deaths, he wrote the song, "It Is Well with my Soul." Notice the lyrics.

When peace, like a river, attendeth my way,
When sorrows like sea billows roll;
Whatever my lot, Thou hast taught me to say,
It is well, it is well with my soul.

Refrain:
It is well (it is well)
with my soul (with my soul),
It is well, it is well with my soul.

The Balance

Though Satan should buffet,
though trials should come,
Let this blest assurance control,
That Christ hath regarded my helpless estate,
And hath shed His own blood for my soul.

My sin—oh, the bliss of this glorious thought!—
My sin, not in part but the whole,
Is nailed to the cross, and I bear it no more,
Praise the Lord, praise the Lord, O my soul!

For me, be it Christ, be it Christ hence to live:
If Jordan above me shall roll,
No pang shall be mine, for in death as in life
Thou wilt whisper Thy peace to my soul.

And Lord, haste the day, when the faith shall be sight,
The clouds be rolled back as a scroll;
The trump shall resound, and the Lord shall descend,
Even so, it is well with my soul.

Horatio and his wife later had three more children, one of which died at age three of scarlet fever. It is said that Horatio Spafford eventually died in 1888 in the Middle East, believing he was the Messiah.

Many Christians think mental illness is "bad advertising" when a Christian struggles with it. Awkward and often avoided, the condition can be very embarrassing for the family who has a loved one dealing with it.

The Mayo Clinic refers to mental illness as a wide range of mental health conditions—disorders that affect mood, thought, and behavior. Examples include depression, anxiety disorders, schizophrenia, eating disorders, and addictive behaviors. Many people have a mental health concern from time to time. I have had loved ones who have dealt with mental health issues and friends with loved ones who struggled with these issues, particularly depression, dementia, and eating disorders.

As Christians and ministers, how are we to handle these challenging issues? It is a struggle to deal with or feel qualified to handle them. I am in no way an expert in this area, but hopefully my bringing this topic to the forefront will help others to feel a little more confident when faced with these issues.

Pastor Ken Gurley preached a message about restoration and listed seven areas that the Word says God will restore. As all his sermons, it was a powerful message delivered with the expertise of a skilled surgeon. He listed the seven areas below:

1. Your health (Jeremiah 30:17)
2. Your joy (Psalm 51:12)
3. Your walk with God (Galatians 6:1)
4. Your walls and hedges (Isaiah 58:12)
5. Your damaged soul (Psalm 23:3)
6. Your life (Ruth 4:15)
7. Your lost years (Joel 2:25)

In regard to mental illness, I want to pull five of these promises out since they can specifically be applied to this subject matter. These are the restoration of health, joy, a damaged soul, life, and lost years.

Restore your health

I don't believe that the restoration of health is exclusive of mental health. One of the amazing attributes of God is His eternal nature. We are confined to the very moment or "dot" on the timeline we are living in called the present, a mind-boggling feature of God's physical world. He is eternal and made us to exist in the present. We cannot see into the future or alter what happened in the past due to the fact that we are limited to the present. God can restore something that once was to what is now because He is not limited to the present. He can reach into the past and put something into the present.

> *For I will restore health unto thee, and I will heal thee of thy wounds, saith the LORD; because they called thee an Outcast, saying, This is Zion, whom no man seeketh after* (Jeremiah 30:17).

This verse states some powerful truths.

1. I will restore health, and
2. I will heal you of your wounds. God referred specifically to degrading comments that other nations had made about Israel.

Health and healing were separated in this passage. I believe health refers to the physical. We damage our bodies by the way we live, but God can restore our health and has also given the body a miraculous restoration system. If we change our lifestyle, it is amazing how He can restore our health. Healthy living and physical restoration were discussed in another section of this book.

He will heal our wounds. The Scripture specifically refers to the healing of emotional wounds from being teased. Much mental illness stems from wounds. Sexual abuse, physical abuse, emotional abuse, isolation, teasing, and bullying lead to feelings of worthlessness. The verse says, "They called thee an Outcast," told that no one wanted them. They were considered unwanted, unworthy, worthless, and cast out. Yet Paul said:

> *For God, who commanded the light to shine out of darkness,* hath shined in our hearts, *to give the light of the knowledge of the glory of God in the face of Jesus Christ. But we have* this treasure *in* earthen vessels *that the excellency of the power may be of God, and not of us. We are troubled on every side, yet not distressed; we are perplexed, but not in despair; persecuted, but not forsaken; cast down, but not destroyed* (2 Corinthians 4:6-9, my emphases).

When it seems everything is caving in around us as it was for Israel at the time of Jeremiah, God has it in control. The emotional wounds of the captives, the physical, mental, or sexual abuse that they faced, along with the humiliation and teasing, made them feel worthless. They struggled with depression and worthlessness.

Paul addressed this beautifully in his letter to the Corinthian church. God will deliver and heal. We may feel as if we are soon to be crushed, yet His Spirit will give us light. We need healing before we can find joy.

Restore your joy

Restore to me the joy of Your salvation And sustain me with a willing spirit (Psalm 51:12, NASB).

God also wants to restore joy to our lives. After healing, God can bring renewed joy. He can reach into our lives and bring that joy we had before we were hurt or damaged by others.

Restore your damaged soul

He restores my soul; He leads me in the paths of righteousness For His name's sake (Psalm 23:3, NKJV).

As He restores joy, He can restore our soul. We are body, soul, and spirit (Genesis 2:7), and God wants to restore our souls and prepare them for an eternity with Him. That is why He did what He did on Calvary.

Restore your life

And he shall be unto thee a restorer of thy life, and a nourisher of thine old age: for

thy daughter in law, which loveth thee,
which is better to thee than seven sons,
hath born him (Ruth 4:15).

God is not just concerned about our eternity, but He is also a restorer of our life. Depression and other mental health issues zap the life right out of us. Sometimes they make it impossible to want to exist. Yet God wants to restore life to us. When it seems impossible to continue, God will restore life to us. As He told Paul, "My grace is sufficient for thee." When pain increases, grace increases proportionally.

When you see someone in an extremely difficult situation, you think you could never handle something like that. The truth is that you couldn't. He or she could not either, but God's grace stepped in when that person felt at the end of his or her own strength. But if a similar ordeal ever comes to your life, His grace will pull you through. He will bring you through and restore your life when you think there is nothing left to be restored, when you say, "I am done, I am worthless, I am finished."

After receiving a drink on the cross, Jesus said, "It is finished." This comes from the Greek word *tetelestai*. What is finished? Matthew Henry mentioned some of the areas "it" covers in "it is finished." Every prophecy had been fulfilled, every jot and tittle; the ceremonial law was abolished with the death of the testator; sin and death are finished so that we have a means to overcome the penalty of such; His suffering was finished as He moved to death; and ultimately the work of His purpose, our redemption, was finished.

Isaiah 53:5 says, "But He was wounded for our transgressions, he was bruised for our iniquities: the chastisement of our peace was upon him; and with his stripes we are healed." The NLT renders it, "But he was pierced for our rebellion, crushed for our sins. He was beaten so we could be whole. He was whipped so we could be healed." Jesus voluntarily submitted Himself to the sufferings and shame so that we could be redeemed, made whole, and healed. It is God's will for us not just to be healed but also to be made whole. He desires not just to give us life but to give us life more abundantly, greater than we could even ask or think (John 10:10; Ephesians 3:20).

Restore your lost years

And I will restore to you the years that the locust hath eaten, the cankerworm, and the caterpiller, and the palmerworm, my great army which I sent among you (Joel 2:25).

One of the most amazing restoration promises is God's promise to restore the years. Mental illness can rob years from the lives of those affected, not just those who have the mental illness but those who love people with mental illness. Years of listlessness, isolation, depression, frustration, no gains or goals, just trying to exist are devastating to the patient and the family of the patient. The cost is months and even years of struggle, stress, and lost relationships. God wants to restore those years that were stolen.

Ear, Thumb, and Toe

In July 2017 Pastor Tyler Walea preached a message using the ear, thumb, and toe passages of Scripture in Leviticus. The reasoning of these specific body parts have always perplexed me, and his explanation was quite revelatory. It was also very fitting for this portion of this book, which I was working on at that time.

> *The priest shall take some of the blood of the guilt offering,* and the priest shall put it *on the* lobe of the right ear *of him who is to be cleansed and on the* thumb of his right hand *and on the* big toe of his right foot (Leviticus 14:14, ESV, my emphases).

He discussed the significance of the three body parts to which the blood was applied: the ear to hear, the thumb to grab (representing strength), and the great toe (representing balance). How important it is for us to hear the still, small voice of the Spirit of God! How critical it is for us to understand the joy of the Lord is our strength! And it is vital to have the balance needed in our foundation, portrayed by the great toe on the right foot.

Stability comes from balance. When addressing mental illness, we must recognize that sometimes we just do not have the answers. We can't figure it out. God does not heal every time. As Whit said, we are "stuck with the frailty of our humanness and dependent on the power of God's will and obliged to keep praying hard."

Doctors have developed and discovered medications that alleviate some of the effects of mental illnesses, drugs or herbal supplements that allow the brain to function more normally. I know a godly pastor who is mightily used of the Holy Ghost, but his mother struggled with dementia. She would sneak out of the house at night and go into neighbors' houses. The family would search for her and find her in someone's home, telling them she was being tortured. Doctors prescribed a small pill for her to take daily, and she had a complete turnaround. She now functions pretty much as normal.

Why does God not heal the dementia instead of requiring medication? I wish I knew those answers, especially when it comes to mental illnesses. It is important that we do our best to try to hear the voice of God. At times it is not easy to stop to listen to the voice of God in the midst of so many distractions.

We also need to trust the strength of God. The priests put the blood on the thumb of the right hand to symbolize the strength we need. We have to trust God when He heals and when He does not heal. We also need to stay balanced. Mental illness will throw your world into a blur of challenges, yet Jesus gives us the tools we need to stay balanced in these intense circumstances.

> *And Moses said unto the LORD, See, thou sayest unto me, Bring up this people: and thou hast not let me know whom thou wilt send with me. Yet thou hast said, I know thee by name, and thou hast also found grace in my sight. Now therefore, I pray*

thee, if I have found grace in thy sight, shew me now thy way, that I may know thee, that I may find grace in thy sight: and consider that this nation is thy people. And he said, My presence shall go with thee, and I will give thee rest. And he said unto him, If thy presence go not with me, carry us not up hence. . . . And the LORD said unto Moses, I will do this thing also that thou hast spoken: for thou hast found grace in my sight, and I know thee by name (Exodus 33:12-15, 17).

I guess in the end we have to understand that God does know our name and where we are all the time. No matter how confusing and challenging life becomes, He knows right where we are.

Once while we sat in church, the pastor called for prayer for those struggling. I reflected on my life, and everything was really great. I had no real financial pressure, my family was all healthy and involved in church, and I enjoyed my work and my life. Within a couple of years, mental illness hit our family and everything was turned upside down. A loved one spent months in the hospital hours away, family normality was totally disrupted, and life abruptly got confusing beyond belief. Things weren't good any more but were truly treacherous.

First Peter 5:8 (CEV) says, "Be on your guard and stay awake. Your enemy, the devil, is like a roaring lion, sneaking around to find someone to attack." The enemy of our soul wants to kill, rob, and destroy us. That is why we have to be on our guard and stay awake and alert. At a time when you least expect it, the devil will attack. In Genesis 4:7 God told Cain, "If thou doest not well, sin lieth at the door." Several versions say, "Sin is crouching at the door." The enemy of your soul crouches, waiting patiently for the right moment to attack. If you have a strong relationship with God and keep your ear, thumb, and great toe (hearing, strength, and balance) connected to Him, you can come out on the other side stronger than you were before.

> *Casting down imaginations, and every high thing that exalteth itself against the knowledge of God, and bringing into captivity every thought to the obedience of Christ* (2 Corinthians 10:5).

This is a powerful and needed verse in this context. Our thoughts will lift all kind of thoughts and feelings above the knowledge of God. Our responsibility is to bring every thought into captivity. We can't allow any of our thoughts to ascend higher than our knowledge of God. All thoughts must be aligned with and brought into subjection to the obedience of Christ. This is often easier said than done, but it is necessary because "sin is crouching at the door."

Allowing your thoughts to get out of control is a very dangerous game to play. When our thoughts rise, telling us that we can do more or better without Christ, we have to bring them back into line with the sovereignty of Christ and bring them into obedience.

Paul understood the power of thought and told the Philippian church:

> *And now, dear brothers and sisters, one final thing. Fix your thoughts on what is true, and honorable, and right, and pure, and lovely, and admirable. Think about things that are excellent and worthy of praise. Keep putting into practice all you learned and received from me—everything you heard from me and saw me doing. Then the God of peace will be with you* (Philippians 4:8-9, NLT).

We can bring our thoughts under control. I think some mental illness begins when we allow our thoughts to stray beyond the areas God wants them to go. We don't "make them obey," and then we go too far. If you want God's peace to be with you, you need to control your thoughts and think on those true, honorable, right, pure, and lovely things.

Look at three different versions of the advice that Paul gave Timothy in 2 Timothy 1:7.

> *For God has not given us a spirit of cowardice, but of power, and of love, and of self-control* (Berean Literal Bible).

> *For God has not given us a spirit of timidity, but of power and love and discipline* (NASB).

For God hath not given us the spirit of fear; but of power, and of love, and of a sound mind (KJV).

God has not given us fear, timidity, or cowardice. He has given us power (miraculous ability), love, and a sound mind (self-control or discipline). The enemy attacks us with fear and intimidation, playing on our natural weaknesses, bombarding our minds, and magnifying our failures. All the while God is challenging us to a higher-level thought life. If we can bring our thoughts into obedience and practice self-control and discipline in our thought life, we can be overcomers. That is what He desires for us.

After my experiences with mental illness, I no longer think someone who is really mentally sick can just "think" himself out of it. I do believe God can heal and deliver. I also believe that at times medication is necessary but that sometimes metal illness can be avoided with a disciplined thought life that has been surrendered to God. All the while we have to keep our guard up, or we will fall prey to the enemy that is crouching at the door, ready to attack in our weakest moment.

Identity

And they came to Jericho: and as he went out of Jericho with his disciples and a great number of people, **blind Bartimaeus,** the son of Timaeus, *sat by the highway side begging. And when he heard that it* *was Jesus of Nazareth, he began to cry out, and say, Jesus, thou Son of David, have mercy on me. And many charged him that he should hold his peace: but he cried the more a great deal, Thou Son of David, have mercy on me. And Jesus stood still, and commanded him to be called. And they call the blind man, saying unto him, Be of good comfort, rise; he calleth thee. And he,* casting away his garment, *rose, and came to Jesus. And Jesus answered and said unto him, What wilt thou that I should do unto thee? The blind man said unto him, Lord, that I might receive my sight. And Jesus said unto him,* Go thy way; thy faith hath made thee whole. *And immediately he received his sight, and followed Jesus in the way* (Mark 10:46-52, my emphases).

We call this man blind Bartimaeus, a beggar about whom we know little. Bartimaeus means "the son of Timaeus." Matthew Henry stated that scholars believe the man was blind and the son of a blind man. This makes the case worse and the cure more miraculous. We find many great messages in this account: miraculous healing, wholeness, God's taking the blind who were born of those blind and making them spiritually able to see, and so on. I want to focus on this man's identity.

The outer garment was an identifier, marking him as a beggar. When Jesus called to Bartimaeus, the Bible relates that he "cast away his garment." He came to God with faith, completely expectant that he would no longer need to be identified as a beggar. The identifying garment that had been in the family for generations was not going to be required any longer. When he came to Jesus, he left his garment and came with the expectation of not just being healed of blindness but no longer needing to sustain his life by begging. He was breaking generations of dependency and shame. The teasing and ridicule finally would be over.

One observation I have had in regard to mental illness: The afflicted make it an identity. People have cancer, but they are anorexic. People have heart disease, but they are schizophrenic. This is common with mental illness. The patient is identified by his illness, and it is not just something he is diagnosed with. I think this is significant. I am also sure that just as God changed the identity of a blind beggar, He can alter the identity of those with a mental illness. He is able. If He did it for Bart, He can do it for you. God can create a testimony of the identity change in some who are struggling with a mental illness. As John Newton noted in the hymn, "Amazing Grace," "I once was lost, but now am found; was blind, but now I see." The capability is available not just to be able to see spiritually but to see God's healing power making people whole.

As we close this section, I made a note from a message I heard Vesta Mangun preach on strongholds. She said strongholds can be a mind-set impregnated with hopelessness that causes us to accept as unchangeable which is contrary to the will of God.

That is a powerful understanding if we can grasp it. We decide that something is unchangeable and hopeless, but God desires to see that situation changed. He wants to deliver, but we have a stronghold in our mind telling us it is hopeless and impossible.

That is where we need to trust in the God who "is able to do exceeding abundantly above all that we ask or think." We may have an incredible imagination, but we can limit God by our lack of belief that He can change our reality into His reality.

God is greater than mental illness. He can heal, deliver, and make whole.

> *The LORD hears his people when they call to him for help. He rescues them from all their troubles. The LORD is close to the brokenhearted; he rescues those whose spirits are crushed* (Psalm 34:17-18, NLT).

That is the desire of the Lord! He is Lord over all, even mental illness.

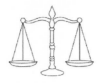

Chapter Seven

Wealth and the Balance

Some may disagree with a section of this book being on finances, but finances play a huge role in our lives. Although money is not spiritual, how we handle money, our attitude toward it, and where we invest our treasure are very spiritual. The Bible discusses finances and possessions more than heaven or hell. It is important to have balance in our finances and possessions as well as having physical, spiritual, and relational balance.

> *Do not lay up for yourselves* treasures on earth, *where moth and rust destroy and where thieves break in and steal; but* lay up for yourselves treasures in heaven, *where neither moth nor rust destroys and where thieves do not break in and steal.* For where your treasure is, there your heart will be also (Matthew 6:19-21, NKJV, my emphases).

Treasure in this verse can be applied to earthly or heavenly treasure. You can really measure the condition of your heart by reviewing your calendar and your checking account. This word, "treasure," can be tied to investment. Where you invest your time and money illustrates the condition of your heart. Where your investment is, there your heart will be! Everyone has treasures. Don't allow temporal things to hold the priority as your most important assets or let things become your security. "Do not invest only in things that depreciate" is sound financial advice, but not investing in temporal things of this world is also sound advice.

Those who know me know that I wholeheartedly believe in the importance of hard work, investing, saving, earning, and giving. Christians should be the best employees a company has. Whatever your hands find to do, you may as well do it with all your might. I often tell younger employees that it doesn't matter what you are technically hired to do. If you agree to work for a company, give it your all, and the reward will come back to you. Work hard. Do your best. Earn a good living. But invest in the eternal. Keep a light grip on finances and the things that moths and rust will corrupt. Instead lay up your investment in heavenly things.

The Bible gives us so much wisdom on how to handle possessions and our finances. We have the greatest instruction manual ever written on the subject on our smart phones and tucked away in our bookshelves, but it does no good if we don't use it to guide our lives. I am going to use this next segment to share some biblical wisdom on finance and possessions.

The righteous will flourish like a palm tree, they will grow like a cedar of Lebanon; planted in the house of the LORD, they will flourish in the courts of our God. They will still bear fruit in old age, they will stay fresh and green, proclaiming, "The LORD is upright; he is my Rock, and there is no wickedness in him" (Psalm 92:12-15, NIV).

I realize that sometimes God calls people into situations that cause them to live in poverty and depend on Him for everything. But I also know the Bible teaches us that His people will prosper and flourish. I am not in favor of a blab-it-and-grab-it prosperity gospel because we are living in a world that is tarnished by sin.

Third John 1:2 says, "Beloved, I wish above all things that thou mayest prosper and be in health, even as thy soul prospereth." God does desire us to be prosperous and in good health. As we prosper spiritually, God also wants us to prosper emotionally, physically, financially, and relationally.

Be sober, be vigilant; because your adversary the devil, as a roaring lion, walketh about, seeking whom he may devour: whom resist stedfast in the faith, knowing that the same afflictions are accomplished in your brethren that are in the world. *But the God of all grace, who hath called us unto his eternal glory by Christ Jesus,*

after that ye have suffered a while, make
you perfect, stablish, strengthen, settle you
(1 Peter 5:8-10, my emphases).

This passage of Scripture gives us a lot of insight and should give us a lot of hope as well. Be alert and aware because our enemy is trying to devour us. Resist him and understand that you are not alone. Others deal with the same things you are dealing with. Because your washing machine breaks down doesn't mean the devil is all over you; it probably just means you had an old washing machine that broke down. They all do. It is all part of the journey. We will go through these things, and as we do, God works on us to mature and establish and settle us through the process.

I believe the equation for success looks something like preparation + opportunity = success. When we prepare ourselves, God will bring the opportunity, and if we have adequately prepared, when that opportunity comes it will be met with success. You cannot wait until the opportunity comes to prepare. You have to prepare in faith that the opportunity will come, and then when it does, success is the result.

Then Moses answered and said, "But suppose they will not believe me or listen to my voice; suppose they say, 'The LORD has not appeared to you.' "
So the LORD said to him, "What is that in your hand?"
He said, "A rod."

*And He said, "Cast it on the ground." So
he cast it on the ground, and it became a
serpent; and Moses fled from it. Then the
LORD said to Moses, "Reach out your
hand and take it by the tail" (and he
reached out his hand and caught it, and it
became a rod in his hand), "that they may
believe that the LORD God of their fathers,
the God of Abraham, the God of Isaac,
and the God of Jacob, has appeared to
you"* (Exodus 4:1-5, NKJV).

The defining question in this story is: What is in
your hand? Moses had left all the pleasures of Egypt, had
escaped to the back side of a desert, and became a shep-
herd. God didn't ask Moses to use something he did not
have. He asked what he had in his hand right then. The
staff Moses carried would be similar to a hammer to a
carpenter or a wrench to a mechanic. It was the primary
tool for his occupation. God wants to take what we have
and turn it into an instrument of His power. He wants to
transform us for His service. It truly is a question of our
approach and attitude toward possessions and money. We
are to be stewards and not owners. A steward is an over-
seer, a commissioner, or a guardian, one who is entrusted
with something.

In his excellent book, *The Stewardship of Life*,
Kirk Nowerly uses the acronym VICTORY to teach us
about stewardship in all areas of life.

V – Vision—If God has given you a vision or
dream, you need to realize that you are the steward of

that vision. Noah, a man who had never seen rain, got the vision of a great flood that would destroy everything on earth. He had to steward the vision to see the ark come to pass. Abraham, married but with no children, received the vision of a great people of whom he would be the father. Spiritual vision enables us to look at life through the eyes of faith, to see things from His perspective.

God usually communicates in less spectacular, though nonetheless supernatural, ways. And though He may not be giving visions to all of us, He gives vision to all of us. He guides us step by step, and sometimes He gives us a vision of what could be, a glimpse into a possibility. Spiritual vision is vital to keeping our eyes on life's ultimate goal. We live in the present, but we must be focused on the future, determined to finish well and see the God-given vision fulfilled in our life.

I – Influence—We are the stewards of our relationships. Everyone has influence, and we should use our influence to draw people toward a relationship with God. Let your light shine. Influence them by living a godly life in front of them.

C – Commitment—We are the stewards of our commitments. Be thoughtful of other people's time by being on time and being prepared when you commit to do something. Make a commitment to your relationship with God by living a balanced life.

T – Time—To God everything in our lives is sacred in the sense that it can be and must be devoted to Him. We must remind ourselves every day that we are spending time. We spend time just like any other commodity. You can never get it back. This is the day that the Lord has made. Are you serving Him or yourself? Whether you are a surgeon or a servant, God sees no difference; whom are you serving? Charles Grisham said that every day he tried to touch God first. Second, he tried to touch a project that will outlive him. Third, he tried to touch people.

O – Opportunity—When we are faced with an opportunity, we are the stewards of that opportunity. In his book, Kirk tells about a friend, Dave, who called and said that he wanted Kirk to go somewhere with him. Where? Germany! "Let's go be a part of the fall of the Berlin wall." Kirk had numerous pastoral duties lined up that week and declined the offer. He regretted being satisfied with the normal instead of the extraordinary once he realized that he had the opportunity to be part of history and turned it down.

> *Be very careful, then, how you live—not as unwise but as wise, making the most of every opportunity, because the days are evil. Therefore do not be foolish, but understand what the Lord's will is* (Ephesians 5:15-17, NIV).

R – Resources—Kirk told an incredible story that I encourage you to read for yourself. In summary, he was left alone on a mountain in Alaska with a tent, a sleeping bag, a gallon jug of water, a lantern, some waterproof matches, a box of granola bars, a hunting knife, a rifle, and five bullets. He quickly ate the granola bars because a plane was supposed to pick him up within a few hours.

He learned a lot about the stewardship of his resources when he sat on the mountain for five days with no news or sight of the plane. He started walking on the sixth day, and that is when he heard the plane.

No matter if you make minimum wage or are the wealthiest man in the world, you have finite resources. It isn't as much about how much you make as about living within your income and resources. You control what you do with what you have; that is stewardship of resources.

Warren Buffet is one of the wealthiest people in the world. He has obviously done well with his finances. He wrote an article about financial advice that was excellent. Some facts about and advice from Mr. Buffet, who has donated over 31 billion dollars to charity:

1) He bought his first share at age eleven, and he now regrets that he started too late! He says things were very cheap at that time. Encourage your children to invest.

2) He bought a small farm at age fourteen with savings from delivering newspapers. He says one can buy many things with few savings. Encourage your children to start some kind of business.

3) He still lives in the three-bedroom house in mid-town Omaha he bought after he married fifty years ago. He has everything he needs in that house. His house does not have a wall or a fence. Do not buy more than you really need, and encourage your children to do and think the same.

4) He drives his own car everywhere and does not have a driver or security people around him. You are what you are. . . .

5) He never travels by private jet although he owns the world's largest private jet company. You should always think how you can accomplish things economically.

6) His company, Berkshire Hathaway, owns sixty-three companies. He writes only one letter each year to the CEOs of these companies, giving them goals for the year. He never holds meetings or calls them on a regular basis. He focuses on assigning the right people the right jobs.

7) He has given his CEOs only two rules:

  1. Do not lose any of your shareholders' money.

  2. Do not forget rule number 1.

  He encourages leaders to set goals and make sure people focus on them.

8) He does not socialize with the high-society crowd. He tells people not to try to show off or put on airs, just to be themselves and do what they enjoy.

9) Warren Buffet does not carry a cell phone, nor does he have a computer on his desk.

10) Bill Gates, the world's richest man, met him for the first time only five years ago. Bill Gates did not think he had anything in common with Warren Buffet. Thus, he had scheduled his meeting for only a half-hour.

But the meeting lasted for ten hours as Bill Gates became a devotee of Warren Buffet.

His advice to young people: Stay away from credit cards and bank loans. Invest in yourself and remember:

A) Money doesn't create man, but man is who created money.
B) Live your life as simply as possible.
C) Don't do what others say. Listen to them, but do what you feel good about.
D) Don't follow brand names; just wear those things in which you feel comfortable.
E) Don't waste your money on unnecessary things; rather, spend on those things you really need.
F) After all, it's your life, so why allow others to rule your life?

Warren Buffet has been an excellent steward of his resources. He has made the most of the resources he has been given and gives some good advice on making the most of your resources. I felt this information was important to share: Stay out of debt, and do not waste money on things you don't need. That is good advice for a balanced life.

Y – You—We are all very limited by ourselves, but Paul said, "I can do all things through Christ which strengtheneth me." We need to be washed in His blood, and we need the power of the Holy Ghost. In myself I do not have much to offer, but with God all things are possible. I know He can take what is in my hand, coupled with the preparation I do by reading and studying, and make something awesome of it.

Finances affect our lives in many ways. The Bible offers wisdom on how to handle our finances. Financial stress is killing a lot of people with too much month and not enough income. The stress on marriages is huge, and the leading cause of divorce is financial pressure. What does the Bible say about money?

> *Do not weary yourself to gain wealth, Cease from your consideration of it. When you set your eyes on it, it is gone. For wealth certainly makes itself wings, Like an eagle that flies toward the heavens* (Proverbs 23:4-5, NASB).

The Bible talks too much about finances for us to isolate this verse. We need to rightly divide the Word to understand this verse's meaning. Jesus told us to take no thought for tomorrow. The sparrows are fed, and we are worth much more than the sparrow. However, in a comparison of other verses, we see that we are to save, not borrow, plan, and prepare.

> *It is better to have little, with fear for the* LORD, *than to have great treasure and inner turmoil* (Proverbs 15:16, NLT).

Proverbs 15:16 brings some balance to Proverbs 23:4-5. When we couple them with what Jesus taught us, we come to the conclusion that the goal is not to ignore your finances or not work but to keep the priorities in balance. If you put your entire focus on gaining wealth but have no peace, you missed the mark. If all you think about is gaining wealth for yourself, you very well may end up realizing that you don't have anything and that what you thought was so important is not really important at all. Plan, work hard, spend less than you make, follow the teachings of the Scripture by seeking first the kingdom of God and His righteousness, and the other stuff will work itself out.

Psalm 37:21 (NASB), "The wicked borrows and does not pay back, But the righteous is gracious and gives." God expects us to be givers. The best thing you can do with money once you put yourself in the position to do so is to be an outrageous giver.

Proverbs 14:23-24 (NLT), "Work brings profit, but mere talk leads to poverty! Wealth is a crown for the wise; the effort of fools yields only foolishness." The Bible does teach us to work hard. God ordained labor in the Garden of Eden when He told Adam "to dress it and to keep it." Some consider work to be a result of sin, but work was originated by God before the Fall.

Discover the overflowing wisdom found in Proverbs 21:5-6, 17, 20. "Good planning and hard work lead to prosperity, but hasty shortcuts lead to poverty. Wealth created by a lying tongue is a vanishing mist and a deadly trap" (NLT). "He who loves pleasure will be a poor man; He who loves wine and oil will not be rich" (NKJV). "The wise have wealth and luxury, but fools spend whatever they get" (NLT).

Proverbs 13:11 (NLT), "Wealth from get-rich-quick schemes quickly disappears; wealth from hard work grows over time." The preacher was talking to us in this verse.

A few more verses to let us know the importance of hard work and the wise handling of our finances.

A hard worker has plenty of food, but a person who chases fantasies ends up in poverty. The trustworthy person will get a rich reward, but a person who wants quick riches will get into trouble (Proverbs 28:19-20, NLT).

I walked by the field of a lazy person, the vineyard of one with no common sense. I saw that it was overgrown with nettles. It was covered with weeds, and its walls were broken down. Then, as I looked and thought about it, I learned this lesson: A little extra sleep, a little more slumber, a little folding of the hands to rest—then poverty will pounce on you like a bandit; scarcity will attack you like an armed robber (Proverbs 24:30-34, NLT).

"Will a man rob God? Yet you have robbed Me! But you say, 'In what way have we robbed You?' In tithes and offerings. You are cursed with a curse, For you have robbed Me, Even this whole nation.

Bring all the tithes into the storehouse, That there may be food in My house, And try Me now in this," Says the LORD of hosts, "If I will not open for you the windows of heaven And pour out for you such blessing That there will not be room enough to receive it. And I will rebuke the devourer for your sakes, So that he will not destroy the fruit of your ground, Nor shall the vine fail to bear fruit for you in the field," Says the LORD of hosts; "And all nations will call you blessed, For you will be a delightful land," Says the LORD of hosts (Malachi 3:8-12, NKJV).

Malachi talked about the devourer. Debt is such a devourer of our finances and our peace. We will find it hard to be balanced when we are strapped with debt and constantly in stress over making ends meet and running out of money before we run out of month.

Just as the rich rule the poor, so the borrower is servant to the lender. . . . Do not agree to guarantee another person's debt or put up security for someone else. If you can't pay it, even your bed will be snatched from under you (Proverbs 22:7, 26-27, NLT).

The *New Living Translation* makes it pretty plain how to handle debt. Unless you want to be a slave, stay out of it. I remember the late Larry Burkett telling the story of a doctor who made great money and wanted to do some investing. His wife wanted to focus on getting out of debt first. They decided to get out of debt first, and within five years he died from cancer. The fact that they were debt-free relieved that burden from his family. Larry Burkett said, "Remember, debt can be an anchor, but it will never be a life preserver."

Dave Ramsey is a nationally syndicated talk-show host and best-selling author whom God has used to help numerous people get out of debt. I strongly recommend his book, *Total Money Makeover*. I wish to share a summary of what he identifies as baby steps for financial health, simple yet effective and based on biblical values.

The baby steps are effective because of the power of focus. The other critical component is a budget. He goes into the details of both in his book. I encourage you to implement his plan. The baby steps are:

A) Save $1,000 fast—This is a baby emergency fund. You will have rainy days and something will happen to your car, your washing machine, or who knows what. But you can't get out of debt if you keep using debt. This $1,000 is to keep you from using debt again.

B) The debt snowball—Cut up all your credit cards and list your debts from smallest to largest. Don't consider the interest rate. Work it like a snowball rolling down a hill. You build momentum when you start with the smallest and then, once that is paid off, work on the next one. Sell stuff, work an extra job, but get intense about getting out of debt. It is more about behavior than it is about math. Stop retirement savings and shave everything from your budget to focus on getting out of debt.

C)   Build an emergency fund—Once out of debt build an emergency fund that consists of three to six months of expenses. This is a big step toward financial peace. Take a moment to imagine your life with no debt and $20,000 in the bank. Sounds peaceful, doesn't it?

D)   Retirement savings—Begin retirement savings again. Start putting 15 percent of your income away for retirement.

E)   College funding—If you have children, begin saving for their college education. This is a huge expense, and if you can help your children get through college without debt, you will do them a tremendous favor.

F)   Pay off your mortgage—Begin to live a little but work to pay off your mortgage.

G)   Build wealth and give—Now you can experience financial freedom. Live like no one else for a while so that later you can live like no one else.

This is a brief description of the baby steps Dave walks people through to help them achieve financial peace. His book will walk you through the steps in a more detailed way. Balance with your finances is critical to living a life with less stress.

I would also like you to imagine being in a service where a missionary presents a need. God deals with your heart. Normally your mind takes you to the fact that you don't have any savings, you are barely making it through the month without running out of money, and you can't afford to give to the need presented. In contrast to that, consider this: You are now debt free, have a nice retirement account, have an emergency fund, and have money in an account set aside for giving. As God tugs at your heart, you can reach for your checkbook and give without hesitation. That is enjoying financial freedom.

As you sit at a restaurant, you see a young family or a military person in the dining room. You discuss with your spouse how nice it would be to pay for their meal anonymously. No problem. That is part of enjoying financial freedom. Save, spend, and give. It is beautiful.

A couple of other thoughts in regard to money. Larry Burkett placed three valuable rules in his book, *Crisis Control in the New Millennium*, and I would like to share them here.

1) Don't risk money you can't afford to lose. Never risk borrowed money.

2) Don't get involved in any venture or investment that you don't understand. Dave Ramsey also stresses this point often. If you can't understand the investment, stay away from it.

3)   Don't make quick decisions. His rule of thumb was that in any decision involving more than $1,000, he waited for at least three weeks. If a decision involved less than $1,000, he waited at least three days. If someone comes to your home to sell you something, he pushes for the sale immediately. Salespeople know that if you take a few days to think about it, they will likely lose the sale because you will realize you really don't need a vacuum cleaner that plays music or a set of knives that can cut a penny. You also realize you don't want another payment on your list. Proverbs 19:2 (NASB) says, "Also it is not good for a person to be without knowledge, and he who hurries his footsteps errs." Proverbs 21:5 (NASB) says, "The plans of the diligent lead surely to advantage, but everyone who is hasty comes surely to poverty." Make sure you understand what you are getting into; take time to think about a decision before jumping into it.

A man with an evil eye hastens after wealth, And does not consider that poverty will come upon him (Proverbs 28:22, NKJV).

By wisdom a house is built, and through understanding it is established; through knowledge its rooms are filled with rare and beautiful treasures (Proverbs 24:3-4, NIV).

Good planning and hard work lead to prosperity, but hasty shortcuts lead to poverty (Proverbs 21:5, NLT).

Plans fail for lack of counsel, but with many advisers they succeed (Proverbs 15:22, NIV).

Planning and godly advice are wonderful when coupled. In your finances, follow the guidelines of the Word and seek some godly counsel from those who have their financial house in order. It will pay great dividends in the long run.

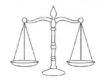

Chapter Eight

Spiritual Occupations

We can learn valuable lessons from the parallel occupations Paul used as illustrations to Timothy.

> *Timothy, my dear son, be strong through the grace that God gives you in Christ Jesus. You have heard me teach things that have been confirmed by many reliable witnesses. Now teach these truths to other trustworthy people who will be able to pass them on to others. Endure suffering along with me, as a good soldier of Christ Jesus. Soldiers don't get tied up in the affairs of civilian life, for then they cannot please the officer who enlisted them. And athletes cannot win the prize unless they follow the rules. And hardworking farmers should be the first to enjoy the fruit of their labor. Think about what I am saying. The*

Lord will help you understand all these things (2 Timothy 2:1-7, NLT).

These verses reveal some attributes that challenge the church to be what God has called us to be. Like so much of the Word of God, this information is inspired for today as much as it was for that day. It can reach into our hearts and give us guidance for our lives.

"Thou therefore, my son, be strong in the grace that is in Christ Jesus" (2 Timothy 2:1). Matthew Henry's commentary talks about 2 Timothy 2:1-7:

> Here Paul encourages Timothy to constancy and perseverance in his work: . . . Observe, Those who have work to do for God must stir up themselves to do it, and strengthen themselves for it. . . . Where there is the truth of grace there must be a labouring after the strength of grace. As our trials increase, we have need to grow stronger and stronger in that which is good; our faith stronger, our resolution stronger, our love to God and Christ stronger. . . . Compare Ephesians 6:10, *Be strong in the Lord, and in the power of his might.*[2]

"And the things that thou hast heard of me among many witnesses, the same commit thou to faithful men, who shall be able to teach others also" (2 Timothy 2:2). Paul was careful as he addressed Timothy here. What you have been given is precious. You don't just throw it out to the swine, as Jesus taught.

> *Give not that which is holy unto the dogs, neither cast ye your pearls before swine, lest they trample them under their feet, and turn again and rend you* (Matthew 7:6).

Yet it is not to be hidden.

> *Ye are the light of the world. A city that is set on an hill cannot be hid. Neither do men light a candle, and put it under a bushel, but on a candlestick; and it giveth light unto all that are in the house. Let your light so shine before men, that they may see your good works, and glorify your Father which is in heaven* (Matthew 5:14-16).

That is why Paul began with the admonition to be strong in the grace that is in Christ Jesus. We need to be strong. The gospel is too precious to handle lightly, and it is too powerful not to handle with care. But we must understand that what we have been given is so precious we must share it. We must not hoard the gospel, but we must grow strong in the gospel and then commit it to those who can share it with others.

This is the method Jesus used. He could have focused on the large crowds and fed millions of people, not just thousands, but He chose to focus the majority of

His ministry on twelve. He chose not the twelve most educated or influential but twelve whom He entrusted to carry the gospel.

> *I have glorified thee on the earth: I have*
> *finished the work which thou gavest me to*
> *do* (John 17:4).

I find it fascinating that before Calvary Jesus said, "I have finished the work." He was not finished, but He had invested His ministry in those who would carry it on. The cross was the place of victory for all of us, but the twelve who had to carry the message beyond the cross needed training. The gospel had to be entrusted to them. That is why Jesus could say He had finished the work.

Edwin Louis Cole was the founder of the men's ministry movement that swept Christianity in the 1990s. He had a slogan, "Teach to teach until every man is taught." His mission was not just to teach men but to teach men to teach others. This reminds me of the saying that you can give a man a fish and feed him for a day or teach a man to fish and feed him for a lifetime. If we want to carry the whole gospel to the whole world, we need to teach to teach and not just teach. We need to guide and grow people rather than just dictating and directing. That is the model Jesus has given us.

Paul continued in the second chapter of 2 Timothy to reveal what he said in the first seven verses.

> *Remember that Jesus Christ of the seed of*
> *David was raised from the dead according*

to my gospel: wherein I suffer trouble, as an evil doer, even unto bonds; but the word of God is not bound (2 Timothy 2:8-9).

He told his spiritual son that this precious gospel is about Jesus. "That is the message I preached to you." Don't ever forget that no matter how successful you are, how famous you become, how much the crowds want something different, Jesus is the essence of everything and needs to be the focal point of everything we do. As J. J. Weeks says in his song, "Let them see You." People need to see Jesus when we sing, speak, or preach. They need to feel Him when we are ministering.

And I, brethren, when I came to you, came not with excellency of speech or of wisdom, declaring unto you the testimony of God. For I determined not to know any thing among you, save Jesus Christ, and him crucified. And I was with you in weakness, and in fear, and in much trembling. And my speech and my preaching was not with enticing words of man's wisdom, but in demonstration of the Spirit and of power: that your faith should not stand in the wisdom of men, but in the power of God (1 Corinthians 2:1-5).

Paul came with the message of Jesus. That was his focus. He wanted Timothy to understand this. Look at the pattern of prayer Jesus taught: "Thy kingdom come. Thy will be done. . . . For thine is the kingdom, and the power, and the glory." It is not about us but about Him. Be strong in the grace. Commit the message to those who are faithful. Are you strong in His grace? Are you faithful enough to carry this precious, powerful gospel?

> *Beloved, when I gave all diligence to write unto you of the common salvation, it was needful for me to write unto you, and exhort you that ye should earnestly contend for the faith which was once delivered unto the saints* (Jude 3).

We must earnestly contend for the faith once delivered to the saints. It is our responsibility to do so.

The above is the background for the spiritual occupations Paul instructed Timothy to consider. Now let's look at these spiritual occupations that Paul introduced to see how they can impact our lives.

The Soldier

> *Endure suffering along with me, as a good soldier of Christ Jesus. Soldiers don't get tied up in the affairs of civilian life, for then they cannot please the officer who enlisted them* (2 Timothy 2:3-4, NLT).

The son of one of our engineers at work just received his wings. To get into the naval academy as a potential fighter pilot, he had to have the best grades, be in great shape, have perfect eyesight, and be almost flawless. Why such high criteria?

A member of the US Navy, he will be assigned to Whidbey Island Naval Air Station near Seattle, Washington. He will fly the F/A-18-G Growler. Why such high standards? Well, the plane costs 60.3 million dollars and is extremely precious and powerful. It has a long list of rockets, bombs, and guns, flies at Mach 1.8, and has a range of twelve hundred miles. The extreme responsibility that comes with such an expensive and deadly piece of equipment requires that only the strongest and most disciplined soldiers get assigned to these planes.

In the chapter that begins this section, Paul stated:

Therefore I endure all things for the elect's sakes, that they may also obtain the salvation which is in Christ Jesus with eternal glory. It is a faithful saying: For if we be dead with him, we shall also live with him: if we suffer, we shall also reign with him: if we deny him, he also will deny us: if we believe not, yet he abideth faithful: he cannot deny himself (2 Timothy 2:10-13).

One of my favorite subjects for reading is World War II. A popular author about this era, whom I enjoy, is Stephen Ambrose. In his book, *A Band of Brothers*, he recaps some of the training the elite 506 Regiment of the 101st Airborne Division paratroopers went through to attain their high status. They were pushed to the limits of their physical and mental abilities. Although it seemed cruel and unnecessary to push the men so hard, once they got into combat, that level of training brought them together as an elite unit.

Private Tipper on the first day of basic training for Easy company—506 Regiment . . .—looked up at Mount Currahee and told someone, "I'll bet that when we finish the training program here, the last thing they'll have us do will be to climb to the top of that mountain." A few minutes later, someone blew a whistle and after they changed they ran up the mountain and back.

After two weeks they were told no running today and taken to the dining hall for a spaghetti dinner, and after stuffing themselves with spaghetti the commander said, "The orders have changed—get ready to run." The entire way up the men were vomiting and they were trailed by ambulances. Anyone who accepted the medics' invitation to ride back in the ambulance was shipped out that same day.

Then on Thanksgiving Day Major Strayer decided it was time for a two-day field exercise. It included long marches, an attack against a defended position, a gas alarm in the middle of the night, and an introduction to K-rations. To make that Thanksgiving even more memorable he stretched wires across a field about eighteen inches above the ground. Machine gunners fired over the top of the wire, and beneath the wire they spread the ground with intestines of freshly slaughtered hogs—hearts, lungs, guts, livers, the works. The men had to crawl through the vile mess like a snake.

Although the men hated these hideous assignments, when interviewed years after the war they credited this for making E company the fighting force it was and admitted that it saved many lives in combat.

1) Train until it becomes second nature.
2) Train until we become one.
3) When in critical situations your training is then automatic.
4) Do what you were programmed to do.

In Holland during the winter of 1944-1945, the men in trenches took a shelling for more than a month in below-zero temperatures. They did not have sufficient winter clothes, had very little rations, and were running out of ammo. These conditions were even worse than their training, but the training had prepared them for this unspeakable hardship. It is likely that the Battle of the Bulge that winter was won because of the extreme training these men had gone through.

II. Paul told Timothy that—1. He must *endure hardness* . . . . 2. The soldiers of Jesus Christ must approve themselves as good soldiers, faithful to their captain, resolute in his cause, and must not give over fighting till *they are made more than conquerors, through him that loved them,* Romans 8:37. 3. Those who would approve themselves good soldiers of Jesus Christ must endure hardness; that is, we must expect it and count upon it in this world, must endure and accustom ourselves to it, and bear it patiently when it comes, and not be moved by it from our integrity.

III. He must not entangle himself in the affairs of this world, v. 4. A soldier, when he has enlisted, leaves his calling, and all the business of it, that he may attend his captain's orders. If we have given up ourselves to be Christ's soldiers, we must sit loose to this world; . . . 1. The great care of a soldier should be to please his general; so the great care of a Christian should be to please Christ, to approve ourselves to him. The way to please him who hath chosen us to be soldiers is not to entangle ourselves with the affairs of this life, but to be free from such entanglements as would hinder us in our holy warfare.[3]

But he that shall endure unto the end, the
same shall be saved (Matthew 24:13).

What a great parallel between our Christian walk
and the training of a soldier! We have to prepare ourselves because hard times and trials will come. We will
experience thorns in our life. We need to be prepared
when that happens.

The Runner

And if a man also strive for masteries, yet
is he not crowned, except he strive lawfully
(2 Timothy 2:5).

Follow the rules. Strive with all that you have.
Never give up. The NLT says it like this, "And athletes
cannot win the prize unless they follow the rules."

I have run in a number of races—5K, 10K, and
half-marathons. I am not that fast and have never entered
a race with the expectation to win. With that said, I am
very competitive. Even when I am just out for a run by
myself, I constantly challenge myself to go farther and
faster even when faced with the reality that I am getting
older and slower. I don't like to drive to run, and I don't
like to pay to run. If I can walk out my front door and go
for a run, it doesn't make sense to me to drive to a park
or a trail. Also, no need to pay for a race when I can run
one every day myself for free. At times it has been nice
knowing I have registered for a race, and I can use that as
motivation if I need it, but usually I just get up and run.

But as I said, I don't expect to win a race. I have placed among the top in my age bracket and usually end up finishing within the first 40 or 50 percent of all runners, quite an accomplishment for me. I finished in the top 40 percent in a half-marathon of over four thousand runners. I try to set a goal of not letting people, whom I pass, pass me later. I also set a goal not to let anyone pass me after about the first mile when the crowd has pretty much got in the groove of their pace. In a half-marathon around mile ten, a lady who had to be twenty years older than I blew right past me. There was absolutely nothing I could do about it. I looked over, and there she was, running right past me. My immediate reaction was "Don't let her pass me!" But my legs just laughed at me as I kept the same pace.

News stories about those who have broken the rules to try to win a race have been rampant in recent years. Some amazing athletes have had titles stripped from them because the knowledge surfaced that they had taken illegal, performance-enhancing drugs. Paul brought to our understanding that our Christian walk is not just about finishing but also about the journey.

My kids used to have a toy Harley-Davidson motorcycle. A button activated the sound of an engine, and the machine would say, "It is not the destination but the journey that matters most." You see, we are in a race, but we have to keep the journey in mind and not just be focused on the destination.

Paul admonished the church at Corinth that we should be "temperate in all things." Be balanced. Don't push the extremes.

Know ye not that they which run in a race run all, but one receiveth the prize? So run, that ye may obtain. And every man that striveth for the mastery is temperate in all things. Now they do it to obtain a corruptible crown; but we an incorruptible. I therefore so run, not as uncertainly; so fight I, not as one that beateth the air: but I keep under my body, and bring it into subjection: lest that by any means, when I have preached to others, I myself should be a castaway (1 Corinthians 9:24-27).

In my "junk" drawer I have a bunch of race bibs reminding me of the races I have run. I kept medals and ribbons and finisher prizes. They are really worthless, just taking up space in my drawer. Even though I was only running for my health and some worthless race bling, I still followed the rules, trained, hydrated, and prepared myself. I followed the rules for a corruptible and meaningless prize.

However, this Christian race is the real deal. We run for an eternal prize. This race is worth running and surely worth keeping our bodies in subjection. The prize is too great to let cares of this world dominate or sidetrack us. We must press on, not looking right or left or allowing distractions from things, lust, status, or sin.

I press toward the mark for the prize of the high calling of God in Christ Jesus (Philippians 3:14).

Wherefore seeing we also are compassed about with so great a cloud of witnesses, let us lay aside every weight, and the sin which doth so easily beset us, and let us run with patience the race that is set before us, looking unto Jesus the author and finisher of our faith; who for the joy that was set before him endured the cross, despising the shame, and is set down at the right hand of the throne of God (Hebrews 12:1-2).

Let's press forward and lay aside the weights and sins that try to pull us off course. We all know what sin is, but this verse also mentions weights. Some things are not sin but are major distractions that pull at us. We can get sidetracked due to these weights that try to derail our spiritual lives. Keep focused on the prize, and don't let the valleys and trials of the journey derail you.

My brother-in-law preached, "What to do when you find yourself in a valley." He talked about prayer and the need to keep fighting, but the focus of the message was "keep moving." As you "walk through the valley of the shadow of death," recall that you weren't designed to live in the valley but to walk through it. Lay aside the weights, look to Jesus, and get through the valley.

The Farmer

The husbandman that laboureth must be first partaker of the fruits (2 Timothy 2:6).

When you first read this verse you think, *Sweet! This one is easy.* After reading about endurance through hardness and the comparison to the struggle of training, this verse seems pretty nice. That is not really the case, though. The verse can also be viewed as: If we want to partake of the fruit, we better labor for the fruit. The old sayings that nothing is free and that you get what you pay for come into play here. Everything has a price. Not only do we labor, but we must exhibit patience and diligence in our labor.

Run with patience the race, patiently labor in the field, and endure hardness. We can see a theme in these spiritual occupations. Before we win the battle, before we get the prize, or before we can partake of the fruit, we have to endure, strive, labor, and never give up.

Do you know what to call a farmer who procrastinates? Bankrupt! Sorry for the bad joke, but seriously, a farmer who waits too long to plant his crop and then tries to cram his work in during the fall will never be a successful farmer. It just doesn't work that way. So the farmer has to be diligent and patient.

This is a powerful glimpse of our lives and the method God uses with us. We have the responsibility to be diligent with preparation but must wait with patience for the time God plans to use us. Success comes when preparation meets opportunity.

Whoso keepeth the fig tree shall eat the fruit thereof: so he that waiteth on his master shall be honoured (Proverbs 27:18).

Or saith he it altogether for our sakes?
For our sakes, no doubt, this is written:
that he that ploweth should plow in hope;
and that he that thresheth in hope should
be partaker of his hope (1 Corinthians
9:10).

This is a great verse. Plow and thresh in hope, and then you can partake of what you hoped for. Don't just hope, but plow and thresh in hope!

Study to shew thyself approved unto God,
a workman that needeth not to be
ashamed, rightly dividing the word of
truth. But shun profane and vain bab-
blings: for they will increase unto more
ungodliness (2 Timothy 2:15-16).

This verse may seem out of place, but it really isn't out of place at all. I enjoy college football and have been a fan of the Ohio State Buckeyes my entire life. The team has what they call "the Grind." Former coach Urban Meyer wrote a great book, entitled *Above the Line*. In this book he talks about instituting what became known as "the Grind." He told his players they would not allow another team to outwork or out-condition them. The Grind is the early morning practices, the extra sessions in the weight room, the extra laps when you are exhausted.

I like to consider 2 Timothy 2:15 as the spiritual grind. Paul taught the younger Timothy that if he wanted to be respected as a spiritual leader, he had to study to show everyone he had paid the price. "You are a workman in the Word. You won't be ashamed, for you have put the time and effort into the Word like a farmer, a runner, or a soldier." No regrets. No looking back. One should exhibit skill at using the Word of God as a skilled surgeon would use a scalpel, using the sharp, two-edged sword of the Word to remove bitterness, hatred, strife, envy, and other sins from the hearts and lives of people.

> *Be patient therefore, brethren, unto the coming of the Lord. Behold, the husbandman waiteth for the precious fruit of the earth, and hath long patience for it, until he receive the early and latter rain. Be ye also patient; stablish your hearts: for the coming of the Lord draweth nigh* (James 5:7-8).

I am not known for my patience. That is something I really struggle with. Yet as a Christian I have to be patient like the farmer. God is patient with us, and we have to be patient with ourselves, souls we reach for, and the wait for His return. He has a pearl of great price for which He gave up everything. We also have a pearl of great price for which we should give up everything!

The soldier, the runner, the farmer—the Christian. Endure hardness, stay committed to Him, show yourself faithful, and never waver or give up. Strive hard, pace yourself, learn the Book, and follow the rules. Learn how to confront the enemy, and finish the course.

Have patience and prepare yourself diligently. Study the Bible. Get into God's Word and grow from it. Establish yourself. These spiritual occupations make up a balanced life.

Motives

All a man's ways seem innocent to him, but motives are weighed by the LORD (Proverbs 16:2, NIV).

This is a critical segment. Many books could be written on the subject of motives. A great line in the Christian movie, *Facing the Giants*, states, "You can't judge yourself on your motives and everyone else on their actions." Since we know our motives it is easy for us to give ourselves the benefit of the doubt, but we have to realize we don't know everyone else's motives. They may have acted wrong with the motive of trying to do well. We have to understand that God knows our motives and weighs them in the balance.

Dig deep into your heart while you strive to keep your motives pure before God. The one with clean hands and a pure heart will be the one who ascends to the hill of the Lord!

Who shall ascend into the hill of the LORD? *or who shall stand in his holy place? He that hath clean hands, and a pure heart; who hath not lifted up his soul unto vanity, nor sworn deceitfully. He shall receive the blessing from the LORD, and righteousness from the God of his salvation. This the generation of them that seek him, that seek thy face, O Jacob. Selah* (Psalm 24:3-6).

This passage contains a powerful promise. Seek the face of the Lord and not just His hands. Seek for His holiness, righteousness, and purity. Seek Him with the pure motive of expanding and cultivating your relationship with Him rather than His gifts or what you expect to receive from your relationship.

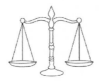

Chapter Nine

To Become

As we come to a close, I encourage you to recognize the power "to become." You can have a balanced, healthy life and still be passionate about God, walk in His ways, and keep His commandments. You can live an overcoming life and have good relationships. It doesn't come easy or even naturally. But it can become a reality.

> *Now as he walked by the sea of Galilee, he saw Simon and Andrew his brother casting a net into the sea: for they were fishers. And Jesus said unto them, Come ye after me, and I will make you **to become** fishers of men. And straightway they forsook their nets, and followed him* (Mark 1:16-18, my emphasis).

The only way "to become" or to receive the "to become" promise involved in the call is to accept the call. When you change and obey, God kicks in and transforms you to something beyond your wildest imagination. Once you accept the call and surrender your will to God, He will do amazing things with your life.

> *What doth it profit, my brethren, though a man say he hath faith, and have not works? can faith save him? . . . Even so faith, if it hath not works, is dead, being alone* (James 2:14, 17).

> *For by grace are ye saved through faith; and that not of yourselves: it is the gift of God: not of works, lest any man should boast* (Ephesians 2:8-9).

> *By whom we have received grace and apostleship, for obedience to the faith among all nations, for his name: among whom are ye also the called of Jesus Christ* (Romans 1:5-6).

> *Know ye not, that to whom ye yield yourselves servants to obey, his servants ye are to whom ye obey; whether of sin unto death, or of obedience unto righteousness?* (Romans 6:16).

I am a math geek. I love equations, calculations, and numbers. Math comes easily to me, and I have always done well in the subject.

To Become

I am not sure if biblical equations are a real thing, but I have come up with some biblical equations I want to share with you.

1.   Faith – Works = Dead
2.   Works – Grace = Pride/sin
3.   Grace – Faith = Wasted Blood
4.   Faith + Grace = Action
5.   Action = Obedience (calling)
6.   Obedience = Servant
7.   New Birth → Christian maturity (New birth is the beginning of a process toward Christian maturity if you stay on the course)

But as many as received him, to them gave he **power to become** *the sons of God, even to them that believe on his name:* which were born, *not of blood, nor of the will of the flesh, nor of the will of man, but* of God (John 1:12-13, my emphases).

What a powerful verse of Scripture! When we are born again, the Holy Ghost gives us the power *to become* the sons of God. We aren't the final product, but we have the power in us to obey, change, be challenged, and be transformed into His image. This is not just about new birth but about new life, the process of becoming more like Him and taking on the attributes of Christ.

In the Gospels we see that multitudes of people followed Jesus (Matthew 4:25). Immediately following this verse we see Jesus begin to teach the Sermon on the Mount. He challenged them with a brand-new approach to live every day. In the day of Roman rule and tyranny, Jesus came with a gospel of peace and forgiveness. Blessed are the poor in spirit, the meek, the hungry and thirsty after righteousness, and peacemakers. Love your enemies, give when no one sees you giving, and forgive unconditionally. Don't just carry the soldier's pack for one mile as required by law, but go further than others are willing to go and do more than others will.

It is amazing that though multitudes followed Him before He taught on self-sacrifice, after the sermon it did not take long before He was alone again. The Beatitudes drove some away. Like the rich young ruler, they followed for the miracles but didn't want the sacrifice. It is hard to become. Not just the destination but the journey matters. The challenge is to become.

> *Now when they saw the boldness of Peter and John, and perceived that they were unlearned and ignorant men, they marvelled; and they took knowledge of them, that they had been with Jesus* (Acts 4:13).

Peter had gone through very trying times. The denial of Jesus, the soldiers in the garden, the ear surgery he tried to perform on the priest's servant, and the "gone fishing" story all took a toll on his commitment and self-confidence. After all that, he had an upper-room experience when the Day of Pentecost was fully come. The power to become entered Peter; he went from the man with the foot-shaped mouth to the apostle who preached the keynote message on the Day of Pentecost. That power *to become* transformed his life.

Character-istics!

Jesus' character in you is the key. He wants us to grow up in Him to the point where people marvel and can't help but notice the power that has transformed our lives. People may see my children and notice they do things that are very similar to things I do. They do them because they have spent time with me. Thus, they repeat some of the things I say and act the way I act at times. When you spend enough quality time with Jesus, you will begin to act like He would act and do what He would do. You start *to become* like Him. The attitudes and actions of Christ become your attitude and actions because you spent time with Him.

> *I beseech you therefore, brethren, by the mercies of God, that you present your bodies a living sacrifice, holy, acceptable to God, which is your reasonable service. And do not be conformed to this world, but be transformed by the renewing of your mind, that you may prove what is that good and acceptable and perfect will of God* (Romans 12:1-2, NKJV).

Transformers are toys that change from a car or a boat into a robot. As you move the parts, they become something similar to what they once were, but they are transformed into something different. This was a fun toy when I was a kid, but it is a good image for us. We are changed from a servant of sin to a servant of righteousness. Once an enemy of God, now we are friends of God.

> *Now the works of the flesh are manifest, which are these; Adultery, fornication, uncleanness, lasciviousness, idolatry, witchcraft, hatred, variance, emulations, wrath, strife, seditions, heresies, envyings, murders, drunkenness, revellings, and such like: of the which I tell you before, as I have also told you in time past, that they which do such things shall not inherit the kingdom of God. But the fruit of the Spirit is love, joy, peace, longsuffering, gentleness, goodness, faith, meekness, temperance: against such there is no law. And they that are Christ's have crucified the flesh with the affections and lusts. If we live in the Spirit, let us also walk in the Spirit. Let us not be desirous of vain glory, provoking one another, envying one another* (Galatians 5:19-26).

> *Nay, ye do wrong, and defraud, and that your brethren. Know ye not that the unrighteous shall not inherit the kingdom of God? Be not deceived: neither fornicators, nor idolaters, nor adulterers, nor*

effeminate, nor abusers of themselves with mankind, nor thieves, nor covetous, nor drunkards, nor revilers, nor extortioners, shall inherit the kingdom of God. And such were some of you: but ye are washed, but ye are sanctified, but ye are justified in the name of the Lord Jesus, and by the Spirit of our God (1 Corinthians 6:8-11).

These passages talk about the works of the flesh. This is where we were. The works of the flesh have dictated our lives. Yet the Holy Ghost is trying to produce in us the fruit of the Spirit. This tug-of-war takes place in our lives. It is as if we have two dogs inside of us, the flesh and the Spirit. Which dog will win the battle of our lives today? The dog you feed is the one that will win. If you feed the flesh, it will win the battle. If you feed the Spirit, it will win the battle. The works of the flesh or the fruit of the Spirit—you have the choice. If you feed your spiritual person you will transform and begin to reflect His image: holy, pure, and righteous.

Howbeit that was not first which is spiritual, but that which is natural; and afterward that which is spiritual. The first man is of the earth, earthy: the second man is the Lord from heaven. As is the earthy, such are they also that are earthy: and as is the heavenly, such are they also that are heavenly. And as we have borne the image of the earthy, we shall also bear the image of the heavenly (1 Corinthians 15:46-49).

This is very similar to the desert detours. Look at Moses, Joseph, or the apostles. They had issues, but a loving God patiently worked on them until they were vessels He could use for His kingdom and glory. The enemy wants to stop you in the process. He wants to destroy your voice. We see in the Gospels that the enemy wanted to kill John the Baptist to stop the voice of repentance. The enemy also wanted to kill Jesus to stop the voice of the miraculous.

Actually, when the people killed Jesus, they didn't stop the voice of the miraculous but rather empowered multitudes to carry the voice of the miraculous. The reason the enemy did not succeed in stopping the voice of the miraculous was because Jesus had empowered people to become the sons of God. They had the rights of the Father at Jesus' death to carry out what He started.

Contrast the prophets whom Obadiah hid from the wicked Jezebel to the apostles in the Book of Acts. We have been ordained to be transformed and to be the voice of the miraculous in our generation, but first we must become fishers of men and sons of God. That was the purpose of Christ's ministry: to develop people to take on His image, to die so that we could be free, and to put His Spirit in us so that we could become the sons of God, taking on His image.

The power to become.

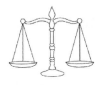

Chapter Ten

Wrapping It Up

When I was growing up, I used to tease my pastor that we never expected him to give an altar call until his third "in closing." I will try to keep the conclusion of this book to no more than three pretty short "in closings"!

The Christian band Building 429 has written and sung some great songs. I was curious why they chose the name, Building 429. Their website reveals they decided upon the name from Paul's writing in Ephesians 4:29, "Let no corrupt communication proceed out of your mouth, but that which is good to the use of edifying, that it may minister grace unto the hearers."

They say, "Quite often the gifts that God gives believers take on an added potency when simmered in the sauce of experience." We learn so much from our life experiences. Dave Ramsey states, "The average person learns from his own experience, the fool doesn't learn from any experience, but the wise person learns from the experience of others." I have met people who had twenty years of experience at life and others who had twenty one-year experiences at life! I want to be the wise person who learns from my own experience and the experiences of others. As every year passes, I hope to learn and grow more and more. I want to learn from the thorns I have put in my life, remove them, and cease to invite any more thorns. I want to be wise and balanced, having priorities in line with God's will and purpose for my life. Proverbs 12:15 (NIV), "The way of a fool seems right to him, but a wise man listens to advice."

Pastor Tyler Walea from First Church in Pearland, Texas, preached a message in October 2016 while I was working on this book. He discussed the importance of strengthening your core. Physical trainers now put a lot of emphasis on strengthening your core. It doesn't matter what sport or type of competition in which you find yourself engaged; your core becomes critically important. When your core is weak, you get off balance. A strong core keeps you in balance. Whether a race-car driver or a football player, an athlete does core exercises. All the running magazines and articles I read talk about core strength and the importance of strengthening your core. But this topic goes far beyond physical core strength.

Pastor Walea explained that a weak spiritual core sets a person's life out of balance. An affair or other slide into sin happens because you have a weak core or weak root system. Then, when you have to reach for a prop because something difficult in life happens, you end up falling. You can't keep your balance because your core is weak. To stay in balance, we need a strong core or a strong root system.

We strengthen our life core by all those things we have discussed in this book. Spiritually, we have to keep our relationship with God strong through prayer, the Word, involvement in a good church, and consistency. Physically, we need to exercise, eat healthy food, and drink plenty of water. Relationally, we need to cultivate our relationships and invest in them. We need a strong root system in all areas of our life to stay in balance.

Finally, some words of advice from the wisest person (aside from Jesus) who ever walked the earth. Solomon said:

> *Don't be too virtuous, and don't be too wise. Why make yourself miserable? Don't be too wicked, and don't be a fool. Why should you die before your time is up? It's good to hold on to the one and not let go of the other, because the one who fears God will be able to avoid both extremes* (Eccelesiastes 7:16-18, GW).

Don't go too far right or too far left, don't focus only on the physical or only on the spiritual, and don't let go of one thing and only pursue another. Fear God, and avoid the extremes of life. Live balanced!

This book is an accumulation of my life's journey, learning, and experience. I hope it is a blessing to you. I am not an expert at any of this "life" stuff. I just work every day at trying to live a balanced life that is pleasing to Jesus. God bless you!

Endnotes

1. http://www.sermoncentral.com/sermons/seven-great-bible-paradoxes-rodelio-mallari-sermon-on-bible-truth-151576.asp

2. *Matthew Henry's Commentary on the Whole Bible*, PC Study Bible Formatted Electronic Database Copyright © 2006 by Biblesoft, Inc. All rights reserved.

3. *Matthew Henry's Commentary.*